RAW INSPIRATION
LIVING DYNAMICALLY
WITH
RAW FOOD

Lisa Montgomery

Martin Pearl Publishing

http//:www.martinpearl.com

Published by
Martin Pearl Publishing
P.O. Box 1441 Dixon, CA 95620
www.martinpearl.com

First Edition: August, 2009

ISBN: 9780981482231
Library of Congress Control Number: 2009928052

PRINTED IN THE UNITED STATES OF AMERICA

10 9 8 7 6 5 4 3 2 1

In memory of Potlucker Sue Roseman

Special thanks to
Raw Chef Dan, Maggie Green, Joel Odhner,Dawn Light and Vito Natale
for the photos of the delicious and georgeous raw dishes.

Hummingbird art work created by Gary Gibbons
Heart Song Mantra by Susan Faucon

Cover Design
Jesse Melchior www.reelmagik.com

Interior Cover and Interior Layout
Jamie Testa & Ariel Rosso

CONTENTS

I am neither doctor nor scientist,
and I don't pretend to be one.
I am a regular person just trying
to find her way through much
research, trial and error.
I am still learning.

In this book, I share
what has worked for me
and for some of my friends.

Don't take my word for it.
Go out and do the research for yourself.
Because what works for me may not work
for you and what works for you
may not work for me.

Plus, as you and your body change,
what works today may not work tomorrow.
The book is meant to be a tool
to inspire you to want to begin living
a healthier and happier way of life.
The choice is yours.
Let today be your first day of
"Living Dynamically."

Lisa Montgomery

MY JOURNEY

WHO ME? WRITE A BOOK?

It's a beautiful June day as I type this introduction to "Raw Inspiration: Living Dynamically with Raw Food." My book is a work in progress just as is my life; its story and my story are not complete.

I hold down a full-time day job as a packaging sales representative. I work 10, 12, 15 hour days in corporate America. My parents are both in their 80's and I devote time to supporting them in their golden years. I own my home and care for two dogs, one puppy, two cats, and one parrot. In spite of my overworked schedule, I am moving in the direction of my true purpose—building my life to fulfill my destiny.

I host monthly raw potlucks in my home that have been blessed with world-renowned guests and speakers such as Viktoras Kulvinskas, Dr. Douglas Graham, Dr. Brian Clement, Dr. Roe Gallo, Victoria Boutenko, Tonya Zavasta, and Paul Nison. I have completed a pilot of a television cooking show "Living Dynamically" that focuses on the raw food lifestyle. I pray one day a television network will pick up this show.

Several people suggested that I write a book about how raw foods changed my life. I thought, "That's fine and well, but I am not a writer. I'm just a regular person—who *really* wants to hear my story?" But, I continued to receive the suggestion from many different people who *did* want to hear my story.

I finally surrendered to the proverbial and divine two-by-four over my head and said "OK, Lord I get it! I'll tell my story about how my life has been transformed by raw foods." I put pen to paper and began writing this book.

When people say they are too busy to pursue their life passions,
my response to them is:
Nonsense, if I can find the time to pursue my life purpose,
you can too!
Make it a priority.
Life is all about choices.
You can get up off the couch and go after your life passion
or you can stay stuck in a job you hate,
with a mate you don't recognize,
in a life that is, frankly, making you miserable.
Or you can take the first step today
towards transforming your physical, emotional, and spiritual life
into your dream life!
It's all up to you; everything in your life starts with you.

Vision is the art of seeing the invisible.
-Jonathan Swift

MY JOURNEY TO RAW FOODS

My journey really began about 15 years ago, the day I signed up for a free spinal exam at my gym. Little did I know that this small action would expand my world and ultimately change the course of my life path.

During the free spinal exam, I was examined by a chiropractor. I knew little about chiropractors at that time. I recalled from my childhood that my father would go to a chiropractor when he was in great pain from a pulled muscle in his back. Going to the chiropractor was not a regular part of my childhood experience. People I knew only went to them as a last resort. The small action of signing up for that exam changed my opinion of chiropractors and ultimately my life. If it weren't for the chiropractor at my gym and the free spinal exam, I would not be where I am today.

I learned from the chiropractor that every vertebrae in your body lines up with a different organ and its function. This information was all new to me. It was just the beginning of what would become a very large learning curve for me, not only physically, but emotionally and spiritually as well. When the chiropractor examined me, he said, "You have bad digestion." I said: "Yes, who told you?" Bad digestion was not, up until that moment, something that I ever discussed with anyone nor even admitted to myself for that matter!

After a series of conversations with the chiropractor and undergoing different food allergy tests with several different doctors, including a homeopathic doctor, I learned that I had candida (a condition attributed to an overgrowth of yeast) and multiple food allergies (dairy, peanuts, and glutens, such as wheat, oat, barley, and rye). This story makes it sound as if my journey through many different doctors was quick and easy. Believe me, it was not! Sifting through, trying to get good sound answers from people who really knew what they were doing was an immense learning experience for me and a long process.

Remember:
Always! It is your choice to take control of your life!
That starts with taking care of
your own emotional, physical, and spiritual health!

If and when you have to or want to get help for a health issue,
persevere until you find knowledgeable people.
Your innate truth will lead you.

I also kept reading everything I could find so that,
in many cases, I knew more than the so-called doctors,
who were supposed to be experts in their field.
It's scary to think, but many of them were not.

Upon learning that I had both candida and multiple food allergies, I was faced with the reality that I had to change my diet to improve my poor digestion and overall health. Because of the candida, I had to avoid foods that would promote fermentation, mold, and continued growth of the yeast, such as white flour, white sugar, caffeinated drinks, fruit, dairy, and mushrooms, to name a few.

Candida is generally caused by antibiotics, birth control pills, and stress. I had been medicated with the birth control pill when I was in a bad marriage and subsequent divorce. I was under great stress from my job and life in general. My food allergies just added another level of complexity to my situation. It was this culmination of life circumstances, one building on another, that led me on this journey that I now share with you.

Your experiences shape your life.
You can grow and learn from your journey
or you can stay stuck in the mud and wallow in your self-pity.
It's all your choice.
Which do you choose?

LIFE-CHANGING CHOICES

Adjusting my diet was a tremendous challenge. Initially, I wallowed in self-pity and felt as though I could not eat anything. To cheer myself up, I went out and bought myself a new place setting of dishes created by a local potter. I love handmade pottery and dishes. I thought that if I couldn't eat anything I wanted, I would at least eat what I could on pretty dishes.

I did a great deal of reading and self-educating to learn what I could and couldn't eat. An employee at my local health food store (Kimberton Whole Foods, Kimberton, Pennsylvania) was a godsend in my life. She gave me a tour of the store and introduced me to a new world of foods that I could eat.

Before this time, I didn't even know what gluten was and now my world was opening up to words like quinoa, millet, and amaranth. By changing my diet, I not only opened my eyes to a whole new world of food, I also opened my world emotionally, physically, and spiritually. To say the change had a huge impact on my life would be an understatement.

Before changing my diet I was mistaking many of the effects of candida and food allergies for 'the normal signs of aging'. In fact, my symptoms had nothing to do with getting older and everything to do with what I was eating. I, like so many other people, did not realize what a huge impact food has on the body—what we eat, how much we eat and when we eat.

I will say many times throughout this book
that once you heal your body physically,
you can then work on your emotional and spiritual growth.
Let's be realistic—if you feel rotten physically,
then you don't care about your relationships with yourself,
your family, your friends, or your Creator/Higher Power.
When you feel rotten, you just exist, barely.
I wanted more than that; don't you?

I grew so passionate about health and nutrition that I decided to become a Certified Holistic Healthcare Practitioner. I enrolled in a weekend program at the Manhattan Institute of Integrative Nutrition (IIN). When I attended IIN, I was already more than 90 percent raw. I tried the different diets while I was a student there so that I could speak from a position of firsthand knowledge, not book knowledge. Other avenues make me physically sick; raw foods make me feel alive and energized. The raw foods lifestyle gives me peace right down to my soul. It resonates with my highest truth.

As part of the curriculum at IIN, we had to work with clients individually. I realized early in the process that even though I had a talent for one-on-one work, I was meant for a bigger venue: teaching, leading, and inspiring larger audiences. Our instructors at IIN asked us what we saw ourselves doing in five years. I wrote in my notebook, "The couple who cooks together stays together." I saw myself as the host of a raw cooking show. And here I am today progressively working toward that very goal.

Once I graduated from IIN, I became 98 percent raw. I say 98 percent and not 100 percent because sometimes I go to a restaurant where something cooked, such as a vegetable, slips into my salad. The week I went 98 percent raw resulted in a funny play of events for me. I had a meeting that week with my "big boss" at the time. After the meeting, I went to one of my coworkers (who is also a friend) and said that it was the best meeting I had ever had with my boss; he was the nicest he had ever been. I also played golf with one of my day job customers at the time and it was the best golf game I had ever had.

Later in the week, I stopped at a local raw restaurant (Arnold's Way in Lansdale, PA) and I shared with Arnold, who is also a close friend, what I had been experiencing all week. I explained that I was calmer, more peaceful, and even feeling euphoric. Arnold pointed out to me that he believes all of the fear, stress, and antibiotics that animals experience as they are raised to be slaughtered on commercial farms is transferred to their meat. This negative energy is then transferred to you when you ingest their meat. Until you stop eating animal you don't realize what a profound effect eating their meat has on you, not only physically, but emotionally and spiritually as well. I was familiar with the concept that it can be bad for you physically to eat animal, that eating meat can contribute to major diseases like heart problems, diabetes and cancer. What shocked me was the impact eliminating meat from my diet had on me spiritually and emotionally.

*A good book regarding the science
behind the impact of eating animals on the human body
is T. Colin Campbell's The China Study.
I also recommend watching the DVD
Healing Cancer From the Inside Out by Mike Anderson.*

A few years ago, after reading every book about raw foods that I could get my hands on, my educational journey into the raw food lifestyle continued. I took my money and vacation time two consecutive years to the Living Light Culinary Institute of Raw Foods in Fort Bragg, California. I became certified as an Associate Raw Chef/Instructor. I have also taken raw cooking classes from local raw chefs and world-renowned chefs such as Juliano, Matthew Kenney, and Raw Chef Dan of Quintessance. I have a friend who has made fun of me because I have taken so many raw food classes. However, all of these classes have helped to prepare me for my own raw cooking show, as well as living my true life purpose of helping and teaching others.

TAKING CARE OF MYSELF FIRST

Once I changed my body, I couldn't, nor did I want to, go back. I learned that eating junk food to make other people feel more comfortable with my new lifestyle would not work. I used to eat a pristine diet and then go to a friend's or to my parents' house for dinner and eat what was served because that was the polite thing to do. But here is the problem: I was the one who was sick the next day.

I now pack my food when I go to my friends' or parents' houses. This way they don't have to figure out what to serve me and I am happy because I don't get sick. The ironic part is that when I start taking out my food, my friends and family start eating my food, too!

Take care of yourself first; you are valuable too!
If you don't care for yourself first
you have nothing to give to anyone else.
And, if taking care of yourself starts with how you eat,
and others feel uncomfortable
because you are eating healthy
and they're eating junk, too bad,
they'll get over it!

You can have a positive impact on other people
just by living your life authentically.
You can set an example by the way you live
and people will come to you and ask why you are so healthy
or why your skin is so nice.
Just live your life authentically and see what happens.

CHEATING

I used to beat myself up when I cheated or inadvertently ate something cooked. Beating yourself up is far more damaging to yourself than having a cooked vegetable every once in a while or cheating on a special occasion. So, if you are going to cheat at a raw foods lifestyle, acknowledge it and move forward with your commitment to your health. When you start to clean up your diet, you will find as I did, that you don't want to cheat anymore. Here's why: before, feeling rotten was normal or so I thought. Now that I feel so good, I don't want to return to feeling rotten. My body wants to be healthy, as does yours. Your cellular structure changes once you eat and live healthfully.

I relate changing your diet to the experience of the recovering alcoholic. You cannot go back. You can choose to pick up that first bite, but you will experience side effects that will make you ill. If you were using food to numb your feelings (in the way that so many alcoholics use alcohol), the problem you were trying to numb still exists, whether you are using the food or not. When you return to using the food, not only do you still have the problem, but now you feel terrible physically, on top of that, and you might be feeling even worse emotionally because you are beating yourself up for your slip.

My question to you is: Is it worth it? My answer for me is: NO. Yes, I am human, and I have cheated. But I get to the point where I stop cheating because the side effects are so bad that it just isn't worth it to me. My ego used to make me think that cooked food would taste so good and I would try it. But it just doesn't taste good to me anymore. You will get to that point, too. Believe me. Hang in there!

The side effects I experience from cheating are not pleasant, to say the least. Within moments, I get a sore throat with lots of mucus. Mucus in the sinuses and throat is an allergic reaction. I now know that my body is trying to tell me something through the mucus; it's not a healthy sign. Another side effect I have when I cheat is that my hands and feet swell up with fluids. I get flu-like symptoms, my digestion gets clogged up and I am totally exhausted. Junk food is truly poison to a healthy body. Now that I am healthy, I recognize this, whereas before, I was blind. Now that my body is no longer accustomed to junk food, my body can't and won't tolerate it. It wants to get rid of the junk food as quickly as possible.

People are poisoning their bodies every day and don't realize it.
If your body fills up with water or your sinuses fill with mucus
recognize that your body is trying to flush out toxins.
Instead of buying drugs to address your symptoms,
look at what you are eating and doing in your life.
Don't buy drugs to mask your symptoms.
Get real with yourself and change!

When I eat cooked food and/or animal meat every orifice in my body gets raw and my bowel movements have an odor. When you go raw, that odor goes away. Try going raw for one week: eat only fruits, vegetables, nuts and seeds—nothing heated over 105 degrees—and then after a week of that diet, eat a cooked meal, and see (or smell!) what I mean.

BUILDING MY RAW FOOD COMMUNITY

Three and a half years ago, I felt there was a need for raw food support and education in my community. To fulfill this need, I started the Living Dynamically Raw Potlucks. Hundreds of raw foodists, and those interested in it, attend the monthly potluck dinners on a regular basis. The potlucks are filled with vibrant energy and have grown to include a truly amazing group of people! We share raw food recipes, techniques and experiences and support each other. World-renowned speakers have even traveled to attend the potlucks at my humble home in Royersford, Pennsylvania. The potlucks truly support raw food enthusiasts in their chosen raw lifestyle.

The potluckers are a group of people who care, share and support one another. Wherever or whenever we meet up with each other in our day-to-day life (not necessarily at a potluck), we are always warmly greeted, supported and cheered on in whatever endeavor we are taking on for the day. It reminds me of how my childhood community was, at least how I perceived it to be. It's like having small town warmth, only it's the raw foodist community.

When I started the monthly raw potlucks, I also started the *Living Dynamically* newsletter and website. The newsletter includes the potluckers' raw food recipes, schedule of the potlucks for the year, biographies and information on upcoming speakers, interesting facts, tips and other information of interest to raw food potluckers and those interested in the raw food lifestyle. Each newsletter is then archived on my website www.livingdynamically.com so people can go back to the website as a reference point.

My natural networking instinct led me to place raw foodist, super model, actress, author and businesswoman Carol Alt on my newsletter distribution list. About three months after I started the potlucks and the newsletter, I was contacted by David Roth, co-writer of Carol Alt's book, *The Raw 50.* As it turns out, Carol was not only receiving and reading my newsletter, she was making the recipes. David informed me that Carol wanted to use several recipes from the *Living Dynamically* newsletter in her upcoming book! One of my recipes and several created by various potluckers are now published in Carol and David's book, *The Raw 50.*

I took this amazing opportunity, speaking with David, and asked if Carol would speak at one of my potlucks. He said that they would make it happen! I started to plan for Carol's visit. I felt that the event should be shared with the larger community in Royersford. I made arrangements for the event to be held at our community park and it took on the name 'The Carol Alt Raw 50 Expo'. A year of planning, preparing and anticipating went into the event with the help and support of countless individuals.

It was finally July 28, 2007, the day of the Carol Alt Raw 50 Health & Nutrition Expo and Carol Alt's celebrity appearance. At 8:00 in the morning, many potluckers arrived at my house to haul supplies to the community park. There were potluckers who were greeters. Others set up the stage, designed floral arrangements, set up chairs for the audience and worked the sound system. We had volunteers who helped in every way imaginable to allow for this event of this magnitude to be such a success. The Expo drew local, state and national politicians, musicians, health and nutrition vendors along with 300 plus attendees. It was a tremendous success.

Thank you to Dick Powell of our local SCORE (Service Corps of Retired Executives) chapter who helped me with publicity and marketing for the event. SCORE's assistance was instrumental in getting local and national media attention. The devoted potluckers made this event the huge success that it was. Their dedicated attendance every month at the potlucks and their help that day was invaluable. I say to all who helped with this event thank you for your love and support, I am eternally grateful.

This good-news story about Carol Alt coming to my hometown
just shows what happens when you open your heart and your home...
Fairy tales do come true!
The success of the Carol Alt Raw 50 Health & Nutrition Expo
is evidence of the benefit that comes from
people working together for the greater good!

TRANSITIONS AMIDST GROWTH

While planning for the Expo, I was still working my corporate day job, working long hours and getting little sleep. During this time, my largest account was purchased and moved to another part of the world. As a result, my income dropped by more than fifty percent. Here I was, in the midst of preparing for the Expo and Carol Alt's appearance, faced with rebuilding my sales territory. I was a scared bunny!

Following the Expo, I continued to work my day job. In March 2008, I became suddenly ill with digestive related problems. I had never before been this sick. I was so sick that I missed three days of work and cancelled a potluck dinner. I was still sick after three days, but forced myself to return to work.

It was a Monday and it turned out to be a horrible day. I was contacted by an 18-year customer who informed me that his corporation could get rebates, also known as "kickbacks", if they went with a national supplier. Despite the longevity of our relationship and outstanding service provided, my colleague was not the decision maker in his company. He was forced to do what the corporation told him to do and switch to the national supplier. I lost that client. I lost another large client that day, as well.

The following day, Tuesday, I was still very sick but I went to work anyway. I went in to one of my customers to take inventory and found that a competitor had "run" my boxes. Here I was still sick and I discovered I was losing yet another customer, making three losses.

I was fit to be tied! I went back to my car and called my boss to tell him what happened. I was so angry. All that my boss said to me was that the company needs more sales. I explained that I had been sick, I was still not well, and I was working 12 to 15 hour days. I asked what more he wanted from me. I nearly shouted into my cellphone. He did not respond.

After that futile conversation with my boss, I cried out to God for an answer. In fact, I remember saying: "Lord, you don't have to take this account from me. You know I'm ready to go. I just don't know how or exactly what it's supposed to look like." I felt like I had hit rock bottom. I wasn't yet aware that my recent illness and the losses at my day job would serve my greater good.

When I first fell sick in March, one of my potluckers commented to me that I take such good care of myself, how could I have become so ill? I said I believed it was a cleansing illness: emotionally, physically, and spiritually. In other words, I believe I was supposed to get sick in order to help me let go of an old way of life. I had to experience this final surrender. It wasn't fun, but necessary.

I called a friend and shared with her my recent trials. Through that conversation and my desperate prayer to God, I gained the strength to take back the reins of my life. I had known for sometime that I wouldn't be selling packaging for the rest of my life and that one day I would be involved in health and nutrition. It was time I sent the message out to the Universe that I was ready to release the old familiar way of life. I was finally ready to pursue my life purpose. At that moment, I was still doing the day job physically, but emotionally and spiritually I had given my notice and moved on. My focus was now fully on the life God intended for me; my life purpose.

Suddenly, I felt much better. I felt as though a huge load was lifted. I'd taken back control of my life. I felt as though the doors of this world and the next had opened up in the grandest manner to show me who I truly was. Now, I would move forward, my sole focus on my true life purpose. I didn't know what that life was going to look like. I knew what some pieces of the puzzle looked like, but I didn't have the whole picture. I moved forward in faith. God started to reveal each detail to me, one divine step at a time.

Two days later, I had an appointment with my chiropractor. The change in my physical body was so dramatic that it was visible and obvious to him. He said he had never seen me smile and glow as I did that day. He could hardly wait to work on me to see if there was a change in the tone of my body, which, of course, there was.

I was learning all of these lessons and letting go of old thoughts, ways, and ideas at the same time I was rebuilding my body physically with my raw foods lifestyle. It was definitely a year of growth! I do not believe it was a mid-life crisis. Instead, I believe it was all about learning who I was and why I was put on this planet.

You can spend the first 35 years of your life being young
and the second 35 years of your life paying for it!
Don't stay stuck—go after your passion and who knows,
Carol Alt may come to your home town!

In one of Joe Vitale's books on manifesting,
he says people think they have to be rich to go after their passion.
But in reality, go after your passion and abundance will come to you.
Please keep in mind that abundance isn't just monetary wealth;
it encompasses emotional, physical, and spiritual well being.

STEPPING INTO THE NOW – MY BOOK, MY TV PILOT

Once I committed to living my highest purpose, I experienced significant shifts in my life. There was a sense of fluidity and synchronicity. I started writing this book. My editor helped me pull it all together and propose it to publishing houses. After sending out proposal and query letters to 20 to 30 publishers and having conversations with four publishers, it was the fourth who published this book. Finding an editor, then a publisher, and continuous editing took more than ten months, which is a relatively short period of time to get a book into print. I have been blessed in that it did not take years and years to bring this book into publication.

I had a creative and brilliant idea for a raw foods cooking show. I connected with a TV producer and we started to work on a television pilot. The market research concluded that 30 percent of Americans are vegetarians with one in every 200 teenagers being vegetarians. At this time, you can view the pilot of Living Dynamically on my website. I must tell you, I have never in my life taken an acting class and had never performed in front of a camera. All the segments were filmed in just two days!

Authentically You

Don't try so hard to fit in when you were born to stand out!
-unknown author

Our schools, our churches, our government and even our society spend so much time trying to make us fit in like sheep, so they can control us—when God intended for us to stand out and let our light shine.

The neat thing about my TV pilot is that I've been told I am a natural. The funny part is that I am just being regular 'ole me, expressing my passion for raw foods, what I learned from all those years of cooking classes, showing my cute gadgets and handmade pottery, sharing my love for my pets and silly stories, telling my silly jokes—it's all me just being me. And that's okay. It is what makes the show entertaining, informative, and most of all, authentic. God wants us to be us—He wants us to use our authentic selves and our natural talents.

God has brought many teachers in to my life. One of my earliest teachers was my aunt who would ask, "Who are you really?" My siblings and I would make fun of her. Now I know what she was really asking! I have two very wise sisters and a brother who have guided me on this spiritual journey. I have also grown tremendously these last few years with the guidance of three teachers: a Native American Indian shaman, a Chinese healer, and a South African spiritual counselor. Everything I have experienced and everyone with whom I have come in contact has helped me to grow and be balanced emotionally, physically, and spiritually.

I am a regular person. I'm not the smartest, I'm not the prettiest, and at five-feet one-inch tall, I'm sure not the tallest. But one thing I have is a burning desire to make a difference in others' lives while I live a life of honesty and integrity. I want to treat people the way I want to be treated. I want to love like God has taught us to love. If all of these statements sound corny or like an overgrown Girl Scout, so be it. They express who I am; I can't be anything different. I spent most of my life being who I was "supposed to be"—the perfect daughter, the perfect wife, the perfect employee.

When you are in conflict with your soul,
you will never be happy.
Take time to be quiet and still with yourself and your God
to find out who you really are and identify your true life purpose.

This book is not only about raw foods, health, and nutrition. These elements are part of this book, but are not all of it. What you put in your mouth has a huge effect on your life, however you will never be healthy emotionally and spiritually without taking care of yourself physically. I hope and pray this book helps you in your life journey as so many people and experiences have helped me.

I have chosen to Live Dynamically.
Won't you start today?
Take the bonbons out of your mouth, get off your butt
and decide to make this the first day of your new dynamic life.
Take back control of your life and Live Dynamically!

PERSONAL STORIES

THOSE WHO HAVE EXPERIENCED THE BENEFITS OF RAW FOOD

I want to express my heartfelt thanks to the beautiful people who have touched my life and for their willingness to share their stories in this book. This section tells the inspiring stories of fellow potluckers and raw foodists. These are stories of recovery, regeneration and hope received from raw inspiration through a raw food lifestyle.

Addiction

If you feel an addictive impulse to indulge in a negative habit, stall until the addictive thought passes. For example: If you feel like indulging in a hot fudge sundae, try drinking a few glasses of water. Many times we think we are hungry or we think we have to eat something when really our body is just thirsty.

In the case of other addictive impulses, while stalling, try substituting a positive distraction such as an exercise, a hobby, or calling a friend. Start cultivating healthy habits such as exercise and maybe your positive habits will outweigh or balance out the unhealthy ones. In time the healthy habits will outweigh your negative habits.

Hey Lisa,

I don't know that you could ever get me to convert to raw foods exclusively but then some of us have the ability to move mountains, one boulder at a time. I see what you have going on and I'm so proud of you. Your heart is in the right place and time.

-JULIE CARVALHO, POTLUCKER

MY FIRST POTLUCK DINNER AT LISA'S
PEGGY O'NEILL, POTLUCKER

My head is still swirling from Saturday night! I so thoroughly enjoyed my first raw potluck dinner. Meeting you and so many vibrant, like-minded people was empowering. Being able to try so many recipes has encouraged me in a way no amount of reading or video watching ever could. Finally, I am convinced that raw meals are completely appealing and satisfying. But most importantly, I won't be so reticent to make many of the recipes for my family and friends.

Thank you for your hospitality. Even your animals emanate the warmth and radiance of your spirit. I look forward to coming with my husband to future dinners. Hopefully, I will become a more active participant. I am certainly willing to help in any way I can.

Raw Vegan, Raw Chef, Opera Singer Loses 170 Pounds on Raw Diet!

Michelle Schulman, Pennsylvania

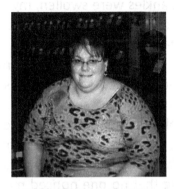

BEFORE 390 lbs...I gained 35 lbs after this, but we don't have any pictures of me when I reached 425 lbs.

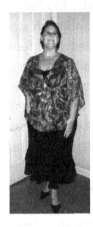

AFTER! A work in progress! 170 lbs lost! From 425 to 255...and still going down!

"I have found NO OTHER WAY to lose weight, <u>keep it off</u> and to control my out of control binge eating than the raw vegan lifestyle!"

On November 14, 2006, my life as I knew it was about to change and it was a change that was *desperately* needed. My life was a painful existence of constant out-of-control binge eating, coupled with the misery of uncontrollable weight gain. That morning, I weighed in at 425 pounds. I'll never forget that last weigh in. I was at the Philadelphia Airport and I snuck the opportunity to weigh myself on a baggage scale when no baggage handlers were looking. I was too heavy for my own scale at home. Aghast at the number on the scale and catching my reflection in the window of the baggage area, I hardly recognized myself. Bloated, swollen, the biggest I had ever gotten, the too-tight size W36 denim jacket I had on wouldn't snap, but it was the only jacket I could get on.

That morning at the airport, I was miserable, desperately yearning to escape my pain, but still caught in an addiction from which I couldn't flee. I was set to fly to San Diego to attend the Optimum Health Institute (OHI), a raw retreat outside of San Diego, California, to turn my life around. I was to make a radical change from a diet of voracious and enormous fast food binges and go on a strict vegan raw food diet. After a tearful farewell to my wonderfully supportive and loving fiancé, Cliff, I rode the escalator up to the flight departure area and was carried further on the conveyer belted walkway, which was fortunate since I could barely walk. My legs, feet, ankles were swollen, my legs rubbed together from friction and each step made my back ache with shooting pains. Short of breath and filled with fear, self-hatred and deep sadness, I wobbled through the airport halls on the verge of tears. My insatiable need to eat found me buying half a dozen deep fried donuts. Bag in hand, I struggled to squeeze myself into a too-small seat in the airport seating area. My misery was palpable. If anyone were to have looked at me kindly or touched my arm, I would have burst into hysterics. Instead, one sad droplet after another flowed from my eyes as I stuffed the sticky glazed confections in my mouth. Filled with self-pity and despair, I cried hoping that no one noticed me crying and knowing not one person there cared about me enough to stop me. I couldn't even stop myself. After the donuts came candy bars, greasy sandwiches, fries, and finally, a fried chicken salad at a sit-down airport restaurant. The tight seat was a constant reminder of my ever growing girth. I pretended I hadn't eaten lunch yet and tried to act nonchalant eating just like everyone else, but who was I fooling? People stared at me in disgust. My disdain for people grew, and the realization of my situation filled me with hopelessness and shame, and the more shame I felt, the more I ate to quell the pain.

On the airplane ride, I sucked up one coke after another, munched continually on cookies and peanuts. Airline meals were downed at precarious risk; the meals could barely sit stable on the tiny table in front of me as my huge stomach and scrunched hips blocked the little table from being able to pull out completely and sit level. My chest was pushed up right under my neck, so I had a hard time breathing and reaching for the food. But even that didn't stop me.

Arriving in San Diego, a taxi drove me to the hotel where I would stay for the night before arriving at the retreat in the morning. After checking into the motel and settling in my room, it wasn't long before I was off in search of food again. The half-block walk from the hotel felt more like painful miles. I was even more bloated after the flight and all that I had eaten, even more filled with shame. In front of the fast food stand, I pretended I was feeding a family and ordered three huge combo meals. It had grown dark and chilly when the food was finally ready. The stuffed bag of food secured in my chubby mitt. It was a twisted mix of excitement to eat the food and self-disgust as I struggled to walk back to the motel. I literally couldn't make it to my room to eat, so I squeezed myself into a poolside chair outside of the hotel which I barely fit into. I was so lonely. I couldn't believe I was so out of control, again, and in the dark, by the pool, all alone, with all of this food. There had to have been over three pounds of food in the take-out boxes. I stuffed myself with the greasy loads of fast food. A disgusted onlooker got up and left, but, by then, I was oblivious, in a food induced daze. I was sickeningly full, and disgusted by the taste of the food, it was really bad. Nevertheless, the fork automatically moved to the food, and then to my mouth, and back again, and again, as if on auto pilot. The beef in the burrito tasted like horse meat and was so foul, yet I kept chewing. My stomach ached and was beyond overstuffed. Bite after disgusting bite, I berated myself. Why couldn't I stop?

Almost three years later, it is still terribly sad to remember how I used to live, how I used to eat, how I used to feel, and how heavy and immobile I was. Most binges were not carried out on foot like that one, but in my car, driving from fast food restaurant to fast food restaurant. I'd eat four or five value meals from different restaurants all in a row. First I'd stop for a double burger, fries, coke and frostie, then drive for another burger, fries, coke and sundae, then to another for a chicken sandwich, fried cheese sticks and a coke, and then to yet another for fried chicken, macaroni and cheese, biscuits, and another coke. I literally couldn't drive past a fast food restaurant without ordering fast food and hamburgers from the drive through. The back of my car looked like a trash heap with bags and messy stinky burger wrappers from my enormous daily binges. And a binge like that...was just lunch. I'd guesstimate I would go on 3,000-5,000 calorie binges, often several times a day. That is how a person gets to weigh 425 pounds.

I had gotten so heavy that I could barely wipe my behind in the bathroom. When a person reaches that level of despair, change is necessary. I knew if I went on like this, I would reach 500 pounds and be one of those people who had to be fork-lifted out of their home.

Life is so different now. After eight months at the raw retreat (I was first a guest and then luckily secured a position as a guest worker in the kitchen), I had lost 140 pounds. After four days of eating raw foods at OHI, my back pains disappeared. I was walking upright with no pain. I followed the retreat diet, ate at raw restaurants a few times a week as a treat, walked and swam as much as I could. It just doesn't call to me anymore. The intense depression and sadness I had carried with me dissipated. I felt reborn and I began to blossom. I lost my insane cravings for fast food and for cooked foods in general. It's been almost three years since I've been raw and I have NEVER once craved another hamburger, or any cooked food for that matter.

At OHI, we not only learned to live the raw life, we learned to embrace health, physically, spiritually and emotionally. I learned better ways to think, cope, and deal with life. Coupled with my new diet, I felt like I had finally been given a life-line, something I could hold onto. I had hope!

After returning home from the retreat, I immediately sought out and secured a job as the raw vegan chef at Arnold's Way Raw Vegetarian Café and Education Center, not far from my home. This was one of those things I now consider "meant to be". Arnold continues to be a huge support to me and a constant teacher and friend. His support has been so crucial to my success!

Un-cooking at Arnold's Way, I thrived on the raw diet, and continued to exercise and lose weight slowly. I had such high energy! But, as time went on, I found I had to refine my raw diet. I was eating a lot of the raw gourmet foods daily in large amounts and doing great, but after about a year of eating very heavily, I found my body in need of a change. I lightened up my raw food choices, and now I prefer to eat a lot of fruit instead, and find my energy skyrocketing again and my body is shedding pounds once again.

The physical changes since going raw have been amazing. Yes, I've lost basically a whole person and know I will continue to lose weight, and fit in chairs wherever I go! I am now able to fit in our bathtub at home and even have room to wiggle around! I love the freedom and mobility that have been restored to me. I can walk faster than my skinny mother AND my normal weight fiancé! I no longer snore. On a scale of 1-10, my snoring was a 15! Now, it's a 0! I no longer stop breathing at night due to sleep apnea. I no longer take medication for acid reflux or suffer from reflux laryngitis, a type of acid reflux that swells the throat and vocal cords and makes it impossible to sing. (When we eat an alkaline raw diet, the body produces very little acid to digest the easily digestible raw food.) My voice soars easily now from low to high and back. I no longer take allergy meds. My skin is clear and flawless and people often marvel, "You have SUCH beautiful skin!" I have very little body odor, too. As a heavy person, I perspired and smelled bad and had bad breath. Now my armpits and my breath are sweet.

Emotionally and spiritually, the changes have been dramatic as well. I'm positive. I'm more direct. I'm empowered to succeed. I believe in myself! I work through my feelings instead of stuffing them. My fiance', Cliff, says I'm calmer, more controlled, and I'm sexier, too! Spiritually, I now feel connected to a power greater than myself.

And since I'm not wasting hours and hours of my life binge eating, I have so much more time to drive to pursue my goals. I sing often and have had newspaper articles written about me and the success I've achieved as a singer and as a raw foodist. I entertain folks often with my opera singing in all kinds of venues, at restaurants, in concerts, in full length operas, at weddings, raw parties, potlucks, special dinners, in churches and temples. I see my gift for singing and my weight loss as a sacred way to connect and communicate with people, to inspire them and to stand as an example of what is possible. I lead weight loss groups, give raw cooking demos, make raw dinner parties (where I sing also!) and give in home raw cooking lessons. My life is now full!

I'm so grateful to my parents for their immense support, and to my fiancé, Cliff, my brother, Ricky, the rest of my family and friends, and my entire "raw family" from OHI and Arnold's Way! Support is crucial!

And, no, I *never* intend to eat cooked food again! The raw vegan diet has kept my out-of-control addiction to food and binge eating at bay when nothing else could. No other diet of the hundreds I had been on, no other therapy, has done this for me. I have *never* lost weight before without immediately regaining it, plus more. I could never stay on a diet! And I never have to again! Raw food is a *lifestyle* that I can live with, blissfully, where I can choose to eat lightly, or treat myself with decadent gourmet fare and feel and look fabulous afterwards! Paradoxically, in being so "extreme", raw foodism is easier than any other diet I've ever been on. Cooked food for me is so intensely stimulating that eating NONE is actually A LOT easier than eating a little. I don't ever want to be that humongous sad girl again who could barely walk. I know if I go back to eating cooked food that I would be as out of control with food as I ever was. I could never stay on a programmed type of diet, a little of this, a little of that. Cooked food for me is an addiction that I'm grateful to be over. I finally feel FREE! So why mess with success?

THE BEAUTY CHEF STORY
JANICE INNELLA, THE BEAUTY CHEF, PENNSYLVANIA

Before I tell my story, I would like to thank Lisa for writing this book. She has been a driving force in the health and wellness community in our area. Her boundless energy and commitment has helped each member in our circle prosper in their goal to live dynamically through raw food.

My background is in the beauty business. Starting as a hair dresser then adding make-up and then skin care and of course food was the final frontier. In the 80's, I first started to notice changes in my health. Ongoing sinus infections, heart burn, weight gain. I was in my early thirties and was not going to take this lying down. I was in the prime of my life and I had just taken on the job of my dreams doing hair and make-up for the Broadway show touring productions of Cats and Phantom of the Opera.

I changed my life style to vegan-vegetarian food by taking macrobiotic cooking classes and started taking care of my health issues at the time. I was introduced to Chinese medicine and Ayurveda. I always tell people I did not survive on the road for nine years on fast food. I had been to every major health food store in the country, traveling on the road from 1989 to 1998.

My health challenge happened when I got off the road in 1998 and moved to Los Angeles, the mecca of the latest and greatest in health, beauty and fitness. I was in heaven, absorbing as many classes and new knowledge as possible. Then, within 6 months, my health started to crash again. I was now 43, another prime time in my life, and I was putting on weight and had no energy. So my next mission was to sort out what was happening to me.

I met a very famous doctor, Dr. Uzzi Reiss. His outlook on health was ahead of its time. I was finally the patient taking notes and learning about my body and my health. He put me on a thyroid medication and later bio-identical hormones. There was still something missing in my diet. I started to eat meat again because a live blood test reported type O and the need to eat lamb and other assorted animal products. Truth be known, I felt good for about three months, but still the weight was not coming off.

FOOD THE FINAL FRONTIER!

I was introduced into raw food at a meeting given by a friend of mine, Arnel Lindgred. He was a fitness expert, trainer, and nutrition expert writing for a healing-focus magazine, which is how I found him. I will never forget eating chocolate pudding made from avocados in the morning on an empty tummy. Wow! did I ever leave on a raw food high. It was so un-believable.

I had to know more about raw food! I read the trusty Healing Retreat magazine and learned there was a school on raw food. The article was about Cheri Soria, who was having a raw food retreat in Oregon. So, after 9-11 when the spa business died and the world was changing, nothing made sense any more. I called the hot springs in Oregon and found out Cheri did traveling retreats and had a home office location in Fort Bragg, in northern California. I signed up immediately with my dear friend Elaine who was my touring buddy and still my dear friend today. We were the health nuts at the time on tour.

Elaine and I headed to northern California where we learned everything there was at that time to know about raw food and why to eat raw. By the end of the retreat, I had lost 10 pounds and had lots of energy. I had not experienced this feeling since my 20's. This was just the beginning of my journey to the mind, body and spirit connection.

I came back and approached the owners of the spa I was working at to put raw food in their healthy organic-cafe. Since they could not cook anything in that location anyway and had the star clientele, I just knew it would work! Having no experience in the food business, I took on this project. I developed all my bread and cracker recipes at that time. At the same time, I was figuring out how to make endless tasty food using a whole new ingredient list, including young coconut, my favorite!

From 2002 to 2003, I had the who's who in Hollywood checking my food out. The film studios were calling every day because I had only a blackboard menu. It was crazy and I soon burned out myself, my waitress and Elaine, who left the road to come help me for no fee, just pure love, and to get the business to the next level. I was changing on so many levels and finding that I really wanted to go back East to my roots, my family, and with my newfound passion.

So, I packed up my car with food processors and blenders and 5 gallon containers of high tech reverse osmosis water and 5 pound bags of nuts and seeds. When I got back to Philly, I started to test market the area. Everyone thought I was from Mars, but they all loved eating my food. I was way ahead of the curve for the Philadelphia area and there were things I needed to learn and be responsible for and be clear about for a real business to sustain me and make a difference in people's lives.

To make ends meet, I stepped back into the beauty world and entertainment field. I started to work on movies locally and did a few other things; private chef and beauty expert on nutrition for a line of skin care products. During this time, I noticed something was happening to me again and I kept thinking it was my thyroid or my hormones. Headaches, energy drops, mood swings, fog brain and a little belly, an insulin resistant sign, although I didn't know this at the time.

I started to drink wheat grass and felt better. Times got tough financially and I was unable to afford what I needed most and had to downsize even more on my life. Finally, a big job came along on a television pilot and another big movie with some great days. That's when it happened! 16-hour days, stress beyond belief. I started to lose weight and became cottonmouth dehydrated and began falling asleep on my feet. It was bad and I did not recover after it was over. How I made it through those weeks, I have no idea.

My brother, who has had diabetes for 39 years, diagnosed me on Christmas Eve, 2007. The family was in a panic because I had a blood sugar count over 400. Adding to the problem, I had no health insurance and was already in debt from difficult times. After that, I looked into a few things to see what help I could get. Finally while at a hospital trying to get a blood test, they suggested I apply for medical assistance. I did, and checked into the ICU. I walked in the day after New Years, 2008.

After three days of being pricked and stuck with needles I had to surrender to the diagnosis. It was my new health opportunity and I would use this to help myself. I believe my life style kept the diabetes at bay, but all the emotional stress and being alone with no partner contributed to an unhealthy life.

Once again, I pulled out all the stops and became a very humble being as I nursed myself back to health. I truly believed I was invincible with raw food and found out that I was human. God became my best friend and I learned a lot about myself and where I fell short with my health and beliefs and taking care of myself. It is not just being thin and looking good. It is the health you radiate from the inside outward. No matter how well you eat, being careless at any age is very damaging.

Drinking fresh juice became the single most key food for me. I did not eat sugar whatsoever and that included no fruit for 6 months. I used berries for blood sugar lows and stevia became my other best friend.

I have become my own specialist with the help of Gabriel Cousins' new book, *There is a Cure for Diabetes,* that came out the month I was diagnosed. My doctor watched how my blood work and numbers kept getting better and better. She said, "You don't need me anymore, keep doing what you are doing and come in for your regular check ups." I knew more about nutrition than the specialist in the class I took to learn about taking insulin and figuring out your food. Since none of my food was in a package, I was on my own, being my own test monkey once again. This time, I was really paying attention to my body and my health. After my last cleanse, I was able to get my insulin shots down to one per day of slow-acting insulin. If I need one or two units for denser food, I take a shot. I can really see how you can get off insulin by just drinking green juices and eating a well-rounded raw diet with some healthy cooked whole grains like brown rice, quinoa, spelt. Using coconut oil to cook with has been a new adventure for me.

I am far from perfect, but I have a lot of information to call on for my daily routine. Eating healthy and raw, exercising, staying connected to my spiritual practice and being in love with my new boyfriend, has manifested a well-rounded healthy "RAW LIFE" for me. I am working on getting my insulin down to zero.

MEET MAUREEN, A FAITHFUL POTLUCKER
MAUREEN MCLELLAN, POTLUCKER

I am fifty-six years old and have had no major health challenges except my inability to keep off excess weight! I have been interested in nutrition and organic gardening for as long as I can remember. Before discovering the raw food way of eating, I had been predominantly eating whole, organic foods. About a year and a half ago, I started reading about the raw food lifestyle. It made sense to me that live and living food would be an even more healthful way to eat. At first, I gradually incorporated more and more raw food into my diet by trying out a new recipe each week. I was amazed that foods I would never have considered eating uncooked tasted so good. I began to really enjoy and look forward to my raw food meals. The recipes were fun to try and cleaning up was so easy. The food was more satisfying. My body seemed to tell me when I had enough to eat, which was a sensation I didn't have with cooked food. And, even though I was eating as much as I wanted, I started to lose weight!

There have been other benefits as well, more noticeably when eating 100% raw food. I have felt an increase in energy and mental clarity, and my skin has become much smoother. While paddling my kayak this summer, I was pleasantly surprised at just how much more flexible my body had become. The 45 pounds I have lost so far has enabled me so much more freedom of movement and it feels wonderful.

Going raw has been a process, a transitioning into a different way of eating and a relearning of some of my beliefs about good nutrition. I have gone through, and enjoyed, two sets of 30 days of being 100% raw, but I am not completely raw all of the time yet. The process of learning about and "becoming more raw" has definitely been an educational, enjoyable, and very rewarding experience.

Cocaine to Coconuts
Joel Odhner
Personal Chef & Nutrition coach
Dr. Oz Files Inner and Outer Beauty, Discovery Health Channel

In 1995, I opened a restaurant that had dinning for 100, a bar, and banquet facilities upstairs that seated 150. We opened first with only dinner offered but within a couple of months we added lunch. I found myself working 100-plus hours a week. This schedule really did not bother me much at the time because I was learning all the different aspects of running the business. So, the hours actually went by quickly for me. Since I did work long hours, I wanted some down time or time to enjoy a beer or two, which obviously contradicted what my wife wanted. This is where you might say the conflict of what I wanted to do and what I should do all began. Time proceeded and I was choosing to stay later to drink more and try a few other unsavory practices.

My priorities got a bit skewed, to say the least. Here I was working about 100-plus hours a week. My then-wife was home with our two daughters. Business was pretty good. I started drinking every day "after" work, though it was never after, since my shift never ended. I was the boss and always on the job. Somewhere around this time, I got turned onto cocaine. This was not my first time. I tried it in college; it was fun, and I did it a couple of times. Customers would give me a line here and there. Finally, I enjoyed it so much that I bought my own and then, of course, I did more and more.

Talk about avoiding life and any responsibility! That was my mission, to pretend I liked being in charge and that I had everything under control. The truth was, I'd much rather be having fun, which in those days meant partying with lots of beer, coke, etc. Looking back at the situation, I now see that I was really hurting; I guess being very unconscious or "not present" led me to make really dumb choices. At the time, it was all about my survival. Trying to survive in a life that was not me or maybe more like a life I thought should be different.

Daily life at the restaurant was so crazy. Looking back, I can hardly believe I actually functioned. Maybe what's even scarier is that so many in our society lead lives that are totally chaotic, and we think it's normal. What is normal? What is the benchmark? Who is doing the right thing? In the many conversations I've had with friends, we all grew up with "normal." Maybe a better response is "this is what I grew up with..." and leave off the judgment of whether it was good or bad; it's just what happened right? We, as humans, seem to love to put judgments on everything that happens or is said. What if we learned to say "is that so" or "that's interesting?" I believe we could have much less drama in our lives by reducing the urge to judge. Life ten years ago in my restaurant was normal, at least to me at the time.

Finally, one fateful night my then-wife told me not to come home and that my stuff would be out front. I tried to call her bluff, but to no avail. I proceeded to go out and do more partying and ended up sleeping in the cab of my pickup on the side of I-95, not my proudest moment, waking up to passing cars. Returning to the restaurant, I saw that Dad was waiting for me and said, "Well, it's time to go and take care of your family". To which I handed him the keys to the restaurant, and called my friend who helped me find a rehab that very next day.

Becoming sober took a lot, and through the support of family and friends, I did. I learned about raw foods about three months into sobriety and I have to say I truly believe it was an integral part of my continuing recovery. In my experience, what raw food did and continues to do is keep me more present or conscious. When I'm in a state of consciousness, life flows. So it is about choices. When you get that which you have chosen, you can change the way you are living to get different results. Really getting the statement "I can choose" is what we call free will. Every day we choose; the core idea here is that a conscious human being is capable of anything. No matter how far down a person falls, there are always choices that can be made which lead to empowered transformation. Choice creates life; no one holds power over you!

What we do is *choose* each and every day, and each choice will have an outcome. What "form" of choice we make will ultimately dictate the "function" of our bodies, emotions, and actions. Knowing that we ourselves alone are totally and completely responsible for our well-being is paramount. Once you take on that level of responsibility, consciousness becomes accessible. No one else is to blame for your life and its outcome; you and you alone are the judge and jury of all emotions you take on, physical challenges you endure and whatever occurs in your life. You create it all.

So within a couple of years, I created Rawlifeline, an online raw food company where we ship meals all over the country. We created events with guests like Dr. Gabriel Cousens, David Wolfe, and Brian Clement, and we sponsored retreats and classes.

Currently, I'm a personal chef supporting people to give their bodies "The Most Powerful Food on the Planet," showing them it can be easy and fun. I also lecture and give classes.

In every moment of our existence we are faced with choices that cultivate who we are. What we choose to fuel our bodies with has an extraordinary impact upon every aspect of our lives. The way we look, feel, and experience our world is interconnected with our source of vitality—the food we eat!

It is my dream to share with you the joy and ease of nourishing your body with the most powerful food on the planet, so you can live your best lives.

Remember my friends, where you find yourself tomorrow is a result of the positive decisions and actions you take today—so make great choices.

MOVING FROM COOKED TO RAW FOODIST
TIMOTHY ARNOLD, POTLUCKER

My wife nudged me into raw food this past year. We ate mostly healthy food, since we were vegetarians. Albeit, I did not think society was ready then and I still am ambivalent, since most believe raw to be a fad. However, we have been 100% raw foodists for nine months and are dedicated to it.

Before converting our eating lifestyle to raw food, my weight had escalated to about 260 pounds and Leslie was 126 pounds. I have been on a yoyo syndrome with my weight all my life between my low of 149 *(for only one day, I could not maintain it)* to my peak of 280 pounds at just five feet ten inches. Today, I now have control over my weight and this is very exciting! As of this writing, Leslie is 105 pounds and I am 165 pounds. Amazingly, I have lost 95 pounds.

In my youth, I ate cooked food and would run. My body would feel much trauma afterward. Since I have been eating raw food, I do not feel anything traumatic after running and I am not tired in the least. I feel exhilarated! When eating raw, I experience a natural "high" and the running just augments it. Running makes me feel like a kid again and seems like a natural thing to do when you are trim and svelte. It was as if my body made me start running because perhaps it would be similar to dancing for joy! In other words, I wanted to run like the Shakespearian phrase "Out of the abundance of the heart, a man speaks." Maybe my running phrase would be "Out of an abundance of a healthy raw diet becoming youthful and lean, one runs for joy!"

The enzymes live in raw food and they die when they are cooked. Pasteurization is a boiling process that destroys enzymes, as well as homogenization of milk, another boiling process. Milk gets boiled twice to make it really good and dead. Our bodies feel lively, as if to dance, when we exclude these boiling processes and eat food in their natural, raw state with all their natural enzymes.

Taste was another issue in our raw transition. Two weeks into our raw diet, Leslie and I revealed to each other that before starting raw, food had become tasteless and boring. But after just two weeks, our taste buds had blossomed and eating was an inspiration of taste, to say the least. It was ecstatic! And still is. That is one factor which will augment one's dedication to 100% raw. Since we had no health issues, the taste factor is good support for remaining dedicated to 100% raw. Man needs discipline whilst eliminating excuses for being lazy. Get off the couch and away from the television. I have been very lazy at times in my life and it was hard to move the body. Sometimes you have to force lethargy, but not always. Rest is good sometimes.

Those who ask how we get protein must understand that, amino acids, the basis of protein, are in all fruits and vegetables. So many myths exist in the cooked food world. True, we have been cooking food for years, but I believe old writings state that during ancient times people initially were raw foodists.

Being a big eater before, I was very surprised that my appetite decreased considerably by eating raw. I do not deprive myself. Dieting is simply "deprivation" and no fun, as most would agree. It is a struggle to diet and I hated it. One must justify depriving themselves and mental trauma ensues. It is battle with the self, usually won by food and ingesting it to the point of stuffing one's face. Food was my friend for a long time and I couldn't get enough of it. Still, I had some restraint because I could have easily been 400 pounds as we see many people today. For those of us who were young in the 1950s and 1960s, fat people were unusual and talked about behind their backs. The usual line was "they must have a glandular problem." Now, it is accepted that 65% of Americans are obese; we are the number one country with this problem. We take for granted obesity as a social norm to the ended whisperings of the so-called "glandular problem" in the past. The Greeks emitted the same whisperings before being conquered.

Our short life expectancy is more nonsense, especially since I have been taught that the physical body can last until 144 years of age. The point is that we can have the best diet in the world, but if we do not utilize all our energies both within and without *(it is mainly "within" that is the problem)*, no one gets to 144. It is basic physics of the science part of life. The proof is that many raw foodists do not get beyond 80 and 90. I believe the proper inner work is not being done. Without an exact key, you cannot open the door, as we all have experienced. It is that simple. Good luck in your raw food ventures, as it brings rewards not fathomed.

Living Dynamically Raw Potlucks: Opportunities to Learn From Guest Speakers
Dawn Light, Dawn of a New Day, Pennsylvania

I found Lisa's potlucks serendipitously. We were just meant to meet! I love the community around her and the quality of her raw potlucks. I always learn something I can incorporate into my life while meeting some wonderful, like-minded people and sharing some amazing and inventive raw food creations. I'm glad she has these events, since she's introducing me to people I might not have heard of otherwise. She's truly a crusader for the raw food community.

I learned much from the speakers she presented and have reviewed their books and products on my website. Many of the ideas I got from Victoria Boutenko, Tonya Zavasta, and Paul Nison worked well for me, so I incorporated them into my lifestyle. I'm still waiting for the book on the benefits of ice-cold morning dunks that Victoria teased about writing!

I read *Raw Family* by Victoria Boutenko and went to one of her weekend events many years ago. It was amazing to see her again at Lisa's raw potluck and hear how her lifestyle had changed after being raw for more than a decade. Victoria's self-experiments, study, and research have saved all of us from making the same mistakes, while giving us a head start and preventing the downhill slide she and her family experienced and had to recover from. Hearing her talk on greens at Lisa's potluck made me realize just how great a benefit it is to be on Victoria's mailing list and get her most recent discoveries that I might not otherwise read about until they get into one of her books in a few years.

I had actually never heard of Tonya Zavasta and I am so glad I learned about her through Lisa. From Tonya, I learned the link between diet and beauty and so many things I just didn't know about the foods we eat. Her interviews of other successful and beautiful women who reversed illnesses and signs of aging were not only inspiring, but cultivated the new belief in me that I can stay young and beautiful all my life. Her products are just the things for supporting a raw food lifestyle, and she is a shining example herself of what is possible. I think the more we see of people staying young and beautiful, the more we will be able to stay young and beautiful. Maybe we can even find out just how long the Creator intended these bodies to last! The fact that she's taken the raw food lifestyle all the way to the quantum level speaks volumes for the benefits of learning from those who have gone before us such as Tonya and Victoria.

Many people marvel at Lisa's raw events and the number and quality of the speakers who come to teach and share with her raw potluckers. I'm downright impressed. I'm very grateful for Lisa's strength, courage, and determination. Such spirit is an inspiration and a benefit to all who come to know her. I love all the people she has gathered around her and enjoy the raw potlucks immensely. I've learned so much, met so many great people and relished being able to gather with like-minded friends. I've also found the raw potluckers interesting and informative; I've even learned healthy lifestyle perspectives beyond raw foods. Lisa Montgomery's Living Dynamically Raw Potlucks are just wonderful!

In Joy!
REGIN BRADFORD, DETROIT, MICHIGAN
FROM *THE DAILY RAW INSPIRATION* FROM JINJEE,
http://www.TheGardenDiet.com

At just over twenty years of age, I was consistently gaining weight and often feeling depressed. My skin was not clear and I had a host of physical and mental distress. During moments like that, it was hard to figure out exactly what to do. Similar to others in our society, I dealt with conflicting messages of how to achieve health. For example, I saw images of slim people on television holding soda pops. These images were followed by happy families around a dinner table of fast food. Often times, athletes were shown drinking sports drinks. Pills were promoted for weight loss. My idea of health was so often associated with unhealthy behaviors that, at my worst time, I was too confused to know what to do about my own unhealthy state. This is the conflict I dealt with on a consistent basis. I felt loss of control over my body's deterioration, and I did not know how to begin to fix it.

At one point, in a state of despair, I sat on my bed while looking outside of my bedroom window, staring at the sunny day. From the part within myself that still believed I was worth more than I appeared to be, I expressed to God one important belief. I expressed to Him that He is the God who created the beauty in nature and I believe it is in His will that I should have that same beauty, having been created by the same God. Little did I know the statement I uttered that day revealed an important concept, which is to view myself and nature as intertwined. Gradually, I became conscientious of the fact that when I ignore the good things in nature, which the Lord has set on this Earth to nourish us, I ignore the optimal way to be healthy.

Suddenly, as if I were a baby again, I noticed that spanning the Earth are fruits, vegetables, and natural foods, which are here for my benefit. It is not surprising that the more I began to partake of food in its natural state, the more I returned to my own natural state of health.

LOCAL WOMAN CHANGES LIFE FOREVER!
VALERIE BARONE
FROM ARNOLD'S WAY NEWSLETTER, LANSDALE, PENNSYLVANIA MAY 2008

In November 2006, my son Francesco was convinced that the raw vegan diet he had been on had cured him of his asthma. At that time, he had only been completely raw for a few months, but for more than a year prior to that he went raw at the first signs of a cold and had no need for an inhaler or steroids, which had always been a necessity at least twice a year. At the time, I was very overweight and was recovering from knee surgery. My son began trying to talk me into going raw for weight loss. I was sure that if I was capable of staying raw that I would eat too much raw food and continue to be obese. I also believed that since I had been unsuccessful at staying on a regular diet, I would never be able to remain raw. I even told him several times that I would never go raw.

Finally, I decided that I owed it to myself to try since there were also claims of having more energy. New Year's Eve 2006 was my first raw day. I woke up with the beginnings of a cold, which always led to the need for steroids for my breathing. That was 15 and a half months ago and I am still eating the raw vegan way. I have also effortlessly lost 85 pounds and my knees feel great. Food and hunger are no longer the problem they once were. I feel more normal, which I am sure sounds odd since I am so different from others when it comes to eating. Unlike other food plans I stayed on years ago; I do not feel cranky or stressed out about social events. Eating raw, and never straying from it, has freed me from the seductive power of food. I believe that in the same way I have been free of the urge to smoke a cigarette for 29 years, I will remain free of the urge for bread, pizza, desserts and other cooked foods as long as I stay away from them and nourish my body with raw vegetable and fruit foods. I should add that I have had a few colds that I lived through without wheezing and I get well without inhalers or steroids. My son also has not needed an inhaler or steroids; just a steady raw diet of fresh veggies and fruits.

There is a raw cafe called Arnold's Way where I can go and talk with other raw foodies for support. Arnold has classes and speakers and a health food store in addition to the cafe. In fact, it was Arnold who first enlightened my son about the powers of becoming a raw vegan.

Although I always liked vegetables, eating raw sounded awful to me before I started. I guess the body changes what it wants. I hope people don't let their preconceived ideas prevent them from trying the raw vegan way of life. They might be like me; they might love it!

Setting Up Your Raw Kitchen, So You Can Live Dynamically

RAW KITCHEN

Your Raw Food Kitchen, Equipment and Utensils
How to set up your raw kitchen, so you can Live Dynamically

When you set up your raw food kitchen, there are a few pieces of equipment that allow you to live your raw lifestyle more dynamically. After trial and error, I have found the following work best for me.

FOOD PROCESSOR: I prefer my *20-cup Cuisinart*. Yes, I know it's 20 cups, but this way when I make a recipe I don't have to make it in batches. The 20-cup is intended for commercial use, but there is a 14-cup that is more economical in price and works just as well. I bought mine at *Fante's Kitchen Wares Shop* in the Italian Market in Philadelphia, Pennsylvania. Fante's is a family owned business. If you don't live in the Philadelphia area, you can go to Fante's website www.fantes.com to order online or call them at 800-443-2683.

BLENDER: The *Vita-Mix* is my favorite high-powered blender. If you already have a blender, don't go out and buy a new one. Wait until your existing blender dies and then buy a Vita Mix. Vita-Mix is durable and easy to use. Others I know love their *Blendtec* blenders. Go online and shop around for the better price. But for me...it's Vita-Mix.

DEHYDRATOR: I've tried many dehydrators and the *Excalibur 9 tier* is my favorite. Don't waste your time on the 4-tray. Get a 9-tray so you can make several recipes at a time. Also, make sure you buy the *Teflex liner sheets*. Most of the recipes require the sheets.

JUICER: There are so many juicers on the market! Find one that works best for you. My favorite is the *Tribest Green Star Juicer* because it can do everything. However, for juicing citrus, the *Citrus Star* is easy to use and cleans up quickly. You can order a juicer at *Tribest's online store* www.tribestlife.com or place a phone order by calling their toll free number 888-254-7336.

CHOPPING BOARD: Use whatever you prefer, however, it is best to use a different board for a variety of items. For example for those eating meat, use a separate board. This prevents cross contamination. The side that has the trough is for cutting fruit and other items that have juice and the flat side is for vegetables that do not release juice when cutting.

SPIRALIZER: Spiralizers are used to turn zucchini or root vegetables in to noodles (angel hair, spaghetti). Some of the spiralizers come with different blades so you can create different types of vegetable noodles. I use the angel hair blade when making my *Three-Nut Basil Pesto Pasta (p. 142)*. If you love spaghetti and other pasta dishes, you will definitely want to include a spiralizer in your raw kitchen. After eating a raw pasta dish made with spiralized zucchini, you won't miss the cooked pastas. You can also spiralize zucchini and add it to any green salad for a different texture and a different look that makes the salad more appealing to the eye.

MANDOLIN: A mandolin is used when you want to finely slice a vegetable or fruit. When you make *Vito's Ravioli (p. 154)* you will use the mandolin to make the ravioli. When you make raw lasagna you use the mandolin to slice the zucchini to make lasagna noodles.

GRATER: Your kitchen probably already has a grater, so don't go out and buy a new one. Instead of grating cheese with your grater you will grate vegetables, garlic, and ginger.

GLASS OR PLASTIC CONTAINERS WITH LIDS: These are a necessity in a raw food kitchen. You can use any type of canning jar. I prefer to use Ball or Mason jars. Go ahead and reuse items you have purchased in glass jars; no need to toss them out. You will make recipes and need to store contents in either glass or plastic containers. If you don't have containers with lids, you can use plastic wrap over any bowl. When citrus is in season, it is great to juice those oranges and pour the juice in glass jars and then store the juice in the freezer, so you can enjoy fresh squeezed juice all year long!

SPROUTING JARS: I use large Ball jars (quart/half gallon size) and leftover gallon olive jars. I use old mesh cloth or mesh plastic that is used in window screens to seal the top of the jars. You can go to a fabric store to get the mesh cloth or hardware store to purchase the screen. I prefer to use the cloth, so I can wash them in the washing machine. Cut the material in the shape of a circle, large enough to cover the opening, then use a rubberband to hold the mesh on the neck of the jar.

I also have an electric sprouting machine I purchased from Sproutman.

COMPOST CONTAINER: Get a small container with a lid, so you can toss unused and uneaten veggies, fruits and other food in it. I keep my container near the sink on the counter where it is easily accessible when preparing meals. After the container is full or before it begins to smell, I dump the contents into a Compostumbler that I have outside. I make my own compost.

Recyclable Utensils and More made by Zak: Zak makes bowls, smiley face spoons *(see back cover)* and a whole line of assorted dishes made out of recycled plastic. I love the fact that they are recycled and on top of that they are extremely colorful. They also have a children's line of dishes as well. Go to their website www.zakdesigns.com to find a store near you or order directly from their online store and have your order shipped direct to your home.

SPATULAS

SPOONS

KNIVES: The following are a "must have" in my kitchen.

ASIAN CLEAVER: Great for opening young Thai coconuts. I purchased one at my local Asian market. I use this every morning when making smoothies for breakfast.

SMALL PARING KNIFE

CHEF'S KNIFE: My sister, Neale, gave me a chef's knife by Wusthof. It came with a sharpener. I use it every day. She purchased it from William Sonoma.

Head Chefs by Fiesta Products: They make great utensils for kids and for big kids like me. The utensils have bright colors and the handles are formed in shapes of human/people bodies. They even bend like Gumby and have suction cups so they stick to the counter top. These utensils are a great way to get children involved in preparing meals and teaching them how to cook or in my case "uncook". You can visit www.fiestaproducts.com to find out where you can purchase their products.

Basic Raw Food Ingredients

By now you have learned that setting up your life to incorporate raw food is much easier than you thought. You really only have four major food ingredients: fruits, vegetables, nuts and seeds. That alone simplifies life. You will never have to go through 95% of a grocery store ever again...unless you want to wave goodbye to a lifestyle that no longer works for you. Once you start eating raw, you will feel healthier and more energized.

One question people always ask me, **"Where do you get your protein?"** In reality, protein is in everything. Do you know there is more protein in kale than in meat and, besides, it's much easier to digest and better for you? Nuts and seeds are full of protein, especially raw almonds. So fear not, your dietary needs will be met.

Fresh Fruits & Veggies: There are so many to select from. Be sure to include green veggies in your meals each and every day!

Nuts: There are a variety of nuts to choose from, but be sure to purchase raw nuts. I store the nuts in the refrigerator and freezer or in glass or plastic air tight containers. I usually buy nuts in bulk, as it is more economical in price and it saves me from having to take time to go out and purchase them when I want to make something. I always have almonds, cashews, pine nuts, macadamia nuts, Brazil nuts, walnuts and pistachios. You don't have to have all varieties when starting out. I recommend you begin by having unpasteurized almonds and cashews.

SEEDS: I always have **sunflower seeds** and **pumpkin seeds.** I store them the same way as the nuts. There are so many items you can make with seeds and nuts. That is what I love about the raw lifestyle, a lot of variety.

DATES: Not only are they tasty, they are amazingly good for you! I also learned that dates, one of the ingredients I use in almond milk, are full of vitamins and minerals.

YOUNG THAI COCONUTS: When you open a coconut and the meat is pink or purplish, do not use. The meat should be white. The younger coconuts will have soft white flesh and the older coconuts will have a thick, tougher white flesh. I use one young Thai coconut (meat and water) in my smoothie every morning for breakfast. The meat and water can be used in desserts such as raw puddings, pies and even raw mayonnaise. The meat alone can be turned into noodles. If you drink the water, it is as if you are putting an IV in your body. Coconut is that healthy for you!

COCONUT PRODUCTS: coconut water, shredded coconut

SWEETENERS: agave syrup, honey (raw), maple syrup *(not really raw, but many raw food recipes call for maple syrup)* If you choose to use maple syrup, then be sure to buy pure maple syrup, not the brands made with high fructose corn syrup and other ingredients.

SALT: Himalayan pink salt, Celtic Sea Salt

FLAVORINGS: Fresh & dried herbs, spices

CACAO POWDER & NIBS: Some people consider this a super food, others say it is not good for you at all. I'll let you decide if it is good for you. I'm not the scientist.

OILS: coconut oil, raw pumpkin seed oil, cold pressed olive oil (cold pressed means it is raw)

FLAX MEAL: This is the basic ingredient for all dehydrated crackers

SEA VEGETABLES: These are great for getting your nutrients and minerals. They have 10-20 times more usable minerals than vegetables grown on land. They are also low in fat and high in dietary fiber.

Some of my favorite sea vegetables are listed below.

ARAME: Mild in flavor. Soak in water till arame absorbs the water which is about five minutes. Soak/season in wheat free tamari or nama shoyu. Eat in salads or add to other vegetables, grains or burgers.

DULSE: Very salty. This is one of the ingredients in the *Atlantic Crab Cakes* on page 150.

HIZIKI: Probably my favorite sea vegetable. I eat it almost every week. Hiziki, believe it or not, is one of the best sources of calcium available. After soaking Hiziki and pouring off the water, I place it in a bowl. Then, I drizzle a little wheat free tamari and sprinkle finely minced garlic and ginger root over the Hiziki. That's it...serve and eat!

IRISH MOSS: Used as a thickener in smoothies, pates and some desserts.

NORI: Everyone probably recognizes nori as the sheets that sushi is made out of. You can purchase raw nori sheets at many grocery stores. It is usually in the Asian section. *Vibrant Veggie Nori Rolls* on page 155 use nori sheets.

SEA PALM: Probably my second favorite sea vegetable. It grows in the ocean off the northwest coast of California. You can eat it dry. Since I no longer eat potato chips and when I get the crunchy munchies, I eat sea palm. It's salty and crunchy. You can also soak sea palm in water, then pour off the water and incorporate it into your salads.

WAKAME: Is most recognizable because it is one of the ingredients in miso soup. A friend of mine just soaks it in water and/or wheat-free tamari and serves and eats it just like that. It is so tasty. See how simple that is to make.

People think you have to be a brain surgeon to eat healthy,
your life does not have to get overcomplicated
just because you start eating sea vegetables.
Keep it simple.

My Typical Week Eating Raw Food

People often ask me, **"What do you eat in a given week?"**

For those of you who are experienced raw foodies, this section will inform you of what a typical week looks like in my life. For those of you who are new to this way of eating, you will be amazed as to how easy and simple eating raw foods can be. Since I am a busy person, as we all are, the weekly plan has to be simple and easy. However, I do make raw gourmet dishes that take more time, but for day-to-day life it has to be quick, simple and easy. I hope you will like the suggestions I give and that the recipes in this book convince you that the raw food lifestyle is simple, easy and even tasty!

A Typical Morning in My Kitchen

Breakfast for me is very easy. I start every day by juicing my wheat grass in my Tribest Green Star Juicer. Wheat grass is like liquid gold. When people ask, "What's it good for?" the answer is, "Everything!" You will feel so much better physically and you will notice you will be energized.

After I drink my juiced wheat grass, I then make a smoothie. Part of my smoothie-making routine includes assistance from my boy, Tweety, an African grey parrot who sits on his counter perch in the kitchen. In just a bit, you will find out how he helps me.

After consuming my green drink, I pull my Vita Mix blender from under the counter so I can blend up a yummy smoothie. Now I am ready to make a tasty and filling breakfast drink.

To make a delicious smoothie, I have many choices. Each day of the week I can make a different variation. Depending on the season, I can have a berry smoothie, a peach smoothie, a mixed fruit smoothie or even a pina colada smoothie. How's that for starting off?

Here we go. Today's smoothie will consist of three bananas, one Thai coconut and whatever fresh fruit I have—usually what is in season. During the summer months I use frozen fruit. I stay away from frozen fruit in the winter when I am cold, because I have discovered my body has a difficult time getting warm.

Now, it's time for Tweety to assist. I take the tips off the banana and give them to Tweety to eat, instead of tossing them in my compost container. Then, I break open the coconut and scoop out the meat, put it in the blender, and then pour the water in after it. Tweety takes the shell and chews on it. Next, I add all the fruit into the blender. My favorite is to use blueberries, raspberries, pineapple, and peaches. Now that I have all the ingredients in the blender, I whip it up and drink. If I drink the entire blender full, that will sustain me until one or two o'clock in the afternoon, sometimes even later. There are days that I just drink a portion and put the rest in a glass container to drink throughout the day.

Green smoothies are popular and very easy to make. Just toss in three bananas, a handful of greens such as kale, sprouts or collards, an apple, a couple of dates, and the water and meat of a young Thai coconut. Then, whip that up in the blender. You can also make your green smoothie for lunch and/ or dinner. I've been known to make a green smoothie, put it in a Ball/Mason jar, and pack it in my cooler for lunch on the road.

Another breakfast idea, in addition to a smoothie, is to take homemade raw granola and pour raw almond milk over it. Almond milk is a cinch to make. If you have never had fresh, homemade almond milk, you are in for a treat. You may never go out and buy milk of any kind again. Almond milk is so healthy and yummy, too! Be sure to use *really* raw almonds, unpasteurized almonds. You can only get unpasteurized almonds from almond growers.

I tend to make almond milk on Sunday. You can make almond milk every day if you like. Just remember to soak the almonds in water overnight before making your homemade almond milk. (See ***Almond Milk*** recipe on page 96.)

How I Manage the Raw Food Lifestyle?
It seems like so much work!

People have also asked me, **"How do you find the time to prepare raw food meals, such as the pizza and other items that take a lot of time?"**

I prepare most of my meals for the week over the weekend. I stock up on ingredients and make several recipes at a time, so I just have them on hand and don't have to worry about timing. Having a variety of items prepared gets me through the week and then I don't have to make anything if I end up not having the time. All I have to do is just assemble what I am in the mood to eat. Yes, I am a normal person; my work week is busy and can be hectic. So, I have found, if I have food already prepared, it allows me to live dynamically throughout the week.

I tend to use the weekend to make pizza crust and crackers. I take the leftover almond pulp I have collected within the week from the almond milk and make crackers. I make the recipes, assemble the mixture on Teflex dehydrator liner trays and begin the dehydrating process. I mentioned earlier that I usually make a variety of recipes. So, it is not uncommon to have all nine of the tiers in my dehydrator full. By the end of the weekend, I have plenty of pizza crust and crackers. I take the finished pizza crust and crackers and place them in a plastic container or a sealed bag so they stay fresh until I use them. It's easy to prepare a pizza sauce and cheese and then store those items in plastic containers or glass jars in the fridge. I am now prepared and ready to make a variety of pizza during the week. I prefer to assemble pizza each day to prevent the crust from getting soggy. Just pack each item in a separate container and assembly when you're ready to eat!

If you would like to view a demonstration on how to prepare pizza crust, you can go to my website www.livingdynamically.com and view the TV pilot show that features me demonstrating how to make raw pizza. I have also included the *Pizza Crust* recipe from Carol Alt's, *The Raw 50,* on page 147.

Preparing a variety of items over the weekend saves me, literally saves me, during the week, especially when it gets hectic. With a variety of choices in the fridge, it is easy for me to select what I will pack for lunch. Then each morning or evening before, I pack my lunch from what I prepared over the weekend. It's not as complicated as it may seem to live dynamically.

Some of My Favorite Recipes Prepared Over the Weekend

One of my favorite things to make is my *Three-Nut Basil Pesto (p.142)*. After making this recipe, I keep the pesto in a plastic container in the fridge. It will stay fresh ALL week! I could eat this pesto every day, and there are weeks I do eat it every day. There are so many ways I eat this pesto, I just don't get tired of eating it. For example, I toss the pesto with some greens and of course, I add cherry tomatoes. I just love my cherry tomatoes, yes, the ones right out of my garden! I also like to slice up asparagus and dip it in the pesto. I often spiralize zucchini and throw on some freshly chopped cilantro and then throw on a glob of the pesto on top. I mix the pesto, so it covers all the veggies. As you can see, it is very easy to make a meal. Just prepare vegetables of your choice and top with *Three-Nut Basil Pesto*. Mix the items together and you have a tasty meal that is also healthy for you. If you don't like the veggies I suggested, prepare your favorites with plain greens, such as lettuce, and top with the pesto. You can also prepare a variety of veggies and eat them by dipping them in the pesto. It's just yummy as a dip!

During the weekend, I also make a couple of *Pates (p.117-119)*, some *Marinated Mushrooms (p.115)*, and a *Toona Salad (p.145)*. I can mix all of those items up, along with fresh veggies and greens and enjoy different meals throughout the week. It's easy. I just pack the variety I want in my lunch each day.

As a treat, I make something a well-known raw chef's sister taught me when I was taking raw food classes. Fill a bowl with fresh fruit sliced in mouth size pieces and then pour some fresh orange juice to cover the fruit. Make *Cashew Cream (p.168)*, which is easy. Just throw raw cashews, raw honey, and/or agave and vanilla in a blender with enough water so it blends into a wonderful cream. Pour the cream on top of the fruit. Sprinkle with raw almond slivers and raw cacao nibs or cacao powder. This is yummy for breakfast or as a dessert.

I also make **Kale Chips** *(p.112)* and **Cream Cheese** *(p.112)*. Kale chips and cream cheese are so easy to make and they are a great snack to have on hand. Yes, the cream cheese I am talking about is not a dairy product. The recipe is in the *Finger Foods & Dips* section of this book. You will soon find out how easy it is to make. To add variation to the cream cheese, mix in onions and dill. Sometimes, I add in chives and scallions. The cream cheese makes a great dressing on a salad or on top of a veggie burger. It's also a great dip with the kale chips. I also use cream cheese when making nori rolls. This cream cheese can be used in a different way every day of the week, because it is so versatile. Now, you see why I like to make cream cheese and keep it in my fridge.

I love to make a variety of pizza during the week. One of my favorites is what I call a "white pizza." White pizza is famous in the Philadelphia area. It is referred to as white pizza because cream cheese is spread on top of pizza crust, making it white. Of course, I can throw on toppings like sliced tomatoes, avocado, onion, olives, or whatever my heart or stomach desires. If I want a true pizza, I could sprinkle some oregano in the pizza crust mixture before dehydrating to give it an Italian flavor. But I'm on a dill kick, so I put dill in the pizza crust mixture. Then I spread tomato sauce and make a red sauce pizza. If I do not want pizza every day, I take the tomato sauce and use it as a dressing on a salad or on a veggie burger. You see, the raw food lifestyle is very versatile.

Because raw food is so filling, I really don't eat dinner. If I do feel hungry, I usually have one of my green drinks or a glass or two of almond milk blended with dates. This milk is so tasty and filling. But, you will want to make at least one dessert and have it ready and waiting to be devoured during the week.

The **Toona Salad** *(p.145)*, **Three-Nut Basil Pesto Pasta**, and **Cream Cheese** recipes are three of my favorites. They have three different tastes and I can change them up. So have fun making these recipes and live dynamically as you experience this healthy and tasty raw food lifestyle.

My Favorite Drinks

My favorite winter drink is raw almond milk. In the summer, my favorite drink is "juiced" watermelon and cantaloupe in my blender. It's refreshing and extremely healthy and cleansing. In fact, I've been thinking lately of my summer drink; the local grocery story actually had cantaloupes and watermelons this week, so for sure, I will be whipping up that drink. In addition, when people are on a healing-cleansing diet, watermelon juice is recommended, along with green energy soup, wheat grass, and fermented raw foods. So drinking watermelon juice is not only tasty, it is extremely healthy, too.

What You Should Know Before Going Raw

When you transition to a raw food lifestyle, please do it gradually. Don't go raw overnight. That could be too much of a shock to your body. Instead, take it slow and try one, two or even three recipes each week.

There is a saying I am known for repeating, **"You spend the first thirty-five years of your life being young and the second thirty-five years paying for it."** So, if it took this many years to get to this point with your diet, health, and lifestyle, then take time to transition to your new lifestyle.

Please note that I changed my eating lifestyle fifteen years ago. The first change was due to food allergies and candida, and then I went micro biotic, vegetarian, and now raw. It wasn't a planned journey, it just happened that way.

Your body will go through some sort of detoxification period. You can count on that! You can't go from eating a standard American diet one day and then eating healthy and not have your body react. Your body does want to be healthy. For me, the detoxification process felt like flu symptoms. Colonics help to speed up the detoxification. It can last a couple of days to a couple of weeks. However, if you transition gradually, this process will be minimal. Stick with it. It will be worth it.

Eating Out! How?

Eating out raw may sound challenging, but it is easier than you think. The easiest place to eat out is at Japanesse restaurants where you can order a seaweed or other sea vegetable salad. When going to a Mexican restaurant, you can order a salad and have them put on raw salsa and guacamole as your dressing.

It used to be when I would go out to eat I would look at the menu to see what I was in the mood for. Now I look at the menu to see what is on the menu that I can make the least deviations to. For example when I do go to my local Mexican restaurant and order a taco salad, I ask them to hold the shell, sour cream and cheese and replace those items with the salsa and guacamole.

Today, there are more and more people who have food allergies and health limitations, so most restaurants are more willing to accommodate special needs. I remember taking a cooking class at a restaurant 20 years ago and they said that 60% of the people who frequented their restaurant would deviate from the menu. So don't be timid about making sure your needs are met. In my case, because I originally changed my diet because of food allergies and made the change about 15 years ago, it is very easy for me to say I have a food allergy and need my food prepared as requested. I have found the servers go out of their way to double check all of the ingredients that go in the meal I am ordering.

You want going out to eat to be a pleasant experience. Just let your server know what you are not able to eat and you should find that they will be more than willing to accommodate your needs. I have found that the servers are used to these requests and some even have a family member or friend with a health issue and they understand.

Don't Have Time, Here's a Thought...

Whole Foods and organic food stores often get deliveries from raw food companies that deliver prepared meals one day a week. So, if you aren't the type who likes to make food, you can buy your fresh meals already made; besides there are raw delivery services that ship and deliver raw foods to your home. Or, make a date with a friend to go to a local raw food restaurant in your area.

SPROUTING

Sprouting is not as difficult as it seems.

However, you will need

the necessary tools, seeds and time.

It takes anywhere from 2- 5 days to grow sprouts.

There are many ways to sprout.

After reading this section,

I hope you will find that sprouting seeds

does not need to be difficult,

but is, instead,fun and easy.

Why Sprout?

The little sprouts are cute and it's fun to play with food...No that's not the reason why you sprout. **There are benefits to soaking seeds!** Sprouted seeds and beans are high in fiber which helps to clean the colon. Besides, food with fiber is more digestible. Sprouts are living food; therefore they have more life force. They are also high in vitality, full of nutrients and they give you energy. Many people refer to the raw lifestyle as "raw-living foods." Sprouts are why this lifestyle is called "living foods."

How Does One Eat Sprouts?

Any way you like! There are so many ways you can eat your homegrown sprouts. I will list a few. Use your creativity and you will come up with delicious ways to enjoy them.

I just love to make *Lentil Burgers (p.143)*. I was first introduced to this recipe by Nomi Shannon who wrote *The Raw Gourmet*. Nomi has graciously allowed me to include the recipe in this book.

It's not difficult to make these tasty burgers. I begin sprouting lentil and mung beans six days before I make the burgers, usually on a Monday, so the sprouts are ready by Sunday. Often I will just throw the sprouts in a salad with greens and throw a burger on it with a pate. And there are other times I choose to not make burgers with the sprouts and instead make a salad. Yes, sprouts do make a wonderful, light salad. Just add your favorite items to make it heartier.

Loreta's Sprouted Peas, Beans & Lentil Salad on page 132 is another yummy salad I make from sprouts I grow.

What's for Lunch?
Sprouts!

Yum! I have a lot of sprouts, even after I make veggie burgers. So, I'm going to put a handful of sprouts on a plate, add a lentil burger on top of the sprouts and spread some *Three-Nut Basil Pesto (p.142)*on top of the burger. I'll add some sliced cherry tomatoes and finely chopped cilantro. Now that's a meal. Since I have so many sprouts, I'll just pack the same items for tomorrow's lunch for the road. I can also drizzle pumpkin seed oil as a dressing, instead of using the Three-Nut Basil Pesto. Be sure to package items separately to prevent the burger from getting soggy. I don't like eating soggy food!

So you see, there are many variations for using sprouts!

Getting Started

Select the variety of seeds you want to sprout. Spout one variety in each jar. Remove all the seeds that are split, not fully developed and look damaged. You can toss those in your compost pile. Once you collect about two tablespoons of good seeds, rinse them in lukewarm water. On the next pages, I explain two ways to grow sprouts. When I am making Loreta's Peas, Beans and Lentil Salad, I put all three seeds in one sprouting jar.

Remember you are growing raw living food. The reason sprouts get labeled living food is because they are exactly that. As your seeds grow, they will turn into sprouts with energy.

Growing Sprouts in Jars

Needed Items

Seeds
Clean, pure water
Glass Jars: quart, ½ gallon or gallon
Rubberbands
Mesh, cloth, plastic or screen (6-8 inch circle)

1. Place seeds in jar. (See quantity chart on p.72)

2. Place mesh over opening of jar, then use rubberband to secure the mesh around the neck of jar.

3. Cover seeds with water.

4. Place jar on counter, so seeds soak overnight.

5. In the morning, dump the water out of the jar into the sink. Keep mesh and rubberband on jar.

6. Fill the jar with pure, clean water.

7. Swish the water back and forth to rinse, and then pour all of the water in sink.

8. Let jar sit on its side on the counter, then cover the jar with a towel. This will allow seeds to grow in the dark. Be sure jar is in a safe spot, so it does not roll on to the floor. You can use your dish drying rack to hold jars on their side.

9. Rinse seeds two to three times a day by repeating Steps 6-8.

   Once sprouts appear, remove the towel. Continue to rinse two to three times a day until mature. In the case of sunflower seeds, be sure to remove hulls before eating.

Growing Sprouts in Soil

Needed Items
Seeds
Organic compost soil
Cafeteria/lunch trays (2 or more)
Watering can
Heavy weights to put on top tray

1. Put seeds in a bowl and cover with water. Soak overnight.

2. Cover a cafeteria tray with ½ inch of organic compost soil.

3. The next day, spread the soaked seeds over the compost soil.
    No need to cover the seeds with soil.

4. Place another cafeteria tray (inverted) over the tray with the soil and
    seeds. You will need to place a couple of weights or something heavy
    on top of the inverted tray to ensure no light gets in.

5. When the sprouts are strong enough to move the top tray, it is time to
    remove the top tray and place the bottom tray in the sunlight.

6. Water sprouts each day until you are ready to harvest.

Note: You can sprout more than one tray at a time!
You can stack numerous soil-filled and seeded trays on top of each
other. When you are finished filling all of your trays you will leave one
clean tray to place inverted on top of the stack of soil-filled and seeded
trays. Place weights on top of the inverted tray.

The sprouts will actually push the weights off the trays. The trays
will rise because the sprouts are strong. You will know when it is time
to remove the top tray and place the tray with the soil and sprouts
under your grow lights, in your green house, on your window sill or
outside in the sun.

My Favorite Seeds to Sprout in Jars

I have provided a chart of the seeds I like to sprout.

Because sprouts are living, they give you energy after you eat them.

Smaller seeds may take only 5 hours to sprout,
whereas seeds with a harder shell can take up to three days.

It will take a week for sunflower and pea shoots to grow to maturity.

Type of Seed	Quantity of Seeds	Rinse Each Day	Growth Cycle	Length to Harvest
Sunflower	3 Tbsp	2-3 times	2 Days	1-2 inch sprouts 4-6 inch shoots
Mung Beans	3 Tbsp	2-3 times	4-5 Days	2-3 inches
Lentil	3 Tbsp	2-3 times	4-5 Days	1-2 inches
Broccoli	1 Tbsp	2-3 times	4 Days	1 inch
Green Pea	3 Tbsp	2-3 times	4-5 Days	1 inch sprouts 4-6 inch shoots

ELECTRIC SPROUTER

I also use the Sproutman's electric sprouter and grow sunflowers hydroponically. The Electric sprouter waters the sprouts for you. Even though I use the electric sprouter for the sunflower seeds, I still start by soaking them in a jar overnight. In the summertime, I plug my electric sprouter outside using an outdoor electrical outlet so they get natural sunlight. It's amazing how much better they grow outside in the summertime compared to sitting on the window sill. There is NO comparison.

Living Dynamically
in Economically Challenging Times

Through the years, I've tried to live resourcefully.
Save in one area so I can spend in another.
But, there are times when we must live resourcefully.
As I completed this book,
the world entered one of these challenging times.

I started looking for ways I could be
resourceful and creative and at the same time
maintain the quality of life I have been accustomed to.
In fact, I started making a list of all the ways I was resourceful
and that's how this chapter came to fruition.

I want to share the ways I am resourceful
in hopes of helping you.
Ironically, you might think by being resourceful my life is boring
and I'm not doing anything in a down economy.
That's not true!
I don't feel like I'm missing out on anything.
In fact, I'm happier now than I've ever been.
Today, it's almost like a game to figure out how I can
be resourceful in ways I've never been.
I challenge you to look at your life and find new ways to save
that allow you to live in a full, quality way.

This section will take a closer look at how
I live my life resourcefully and at the same time,
I'm living dynamically.

LIVING RESOURCEFULLY

GETTING THE MOST OUT OF RAW FOOD

HOW I KEEP MY FOOD BILL AS LOW AS POSSIBLE!

BUY IN BULK

Yes, buying in bulk costs more upfront, but it saves money in the long run. I've listed a variety of food I purchase in bulk. In some cases, I have included where I get those items.

THAI COCONUTS: I buy young Thai coconuts by the case and it is so much cheaper. I buy a case of coconuts at a time at a local Asian market. I have found coconut prices are more economical at an Asian market, usually half the price compared to a local health store. But, if you don't have an Asian market in your neighborhood, it is still cheaper to buy coconuts by the case at your local market. It makes sense for me to buy coconuts in bulk, since I use one coconut every morning in my smoothie. I go through a lot of coconuts in a year! Begin your search for an Asian market near you!

RAW NUTS: I buy raw nuts in bulk. I found that the cheapest place near me is in Lancaster County. *Millers Natural Products* is a wonderful Amish health store. Their prices are the best in greater Philadelphia and the experience driving out through the farms in Lancaster County is beautiful and peaceful. I stock up on nuts and throw them in the freezer. I just pull them out when I need them. Again, I save on price, time and gas by purchasing in bulk.

RAW UNPASTEURIZED ALMONDS: Be sure to purchase raw "unpasteurized" almonds. Don't be fooled by the labels in the stores stating "raw", because they are not truly raw. California almonds go through a pasteurization process that in turn kills the life out of almonds and prevents them from sprouting. You'll need to find an almond grower that does not pasteurize their almonds, because unpasteurized almonds are not allowed to be sold in stores per a Federal Regulation that was passed in 2007. So, when you visit California, be sure to visit the farmers markets and find an almond farmer.

WHEAT GRASS: I buy wheat grass by the tray. Buying wheat grass already cut costs two to four times more depending on where purchased. As soon as I get home with my tray of wheat grass, I cut the grass by the handfuls and store the cut grass in Ziplock bags that are stored in my refrigerator. This method preserves the grass for a week or two. If I do not cut the grass, it will turn yellow and rot. During the summer, I am able to get a second cutting for every wheat grass tray I purchase. After I cut a portion for my green drink and store the rest in baggies, I place the tray out in the sun and the grass will re-grow.

KALE: I now buy kale by the half case and I save 50 to 75 cents per bundle. That adds up over a month and over the year. I use kale in my salads, green drinks, and I make kale chips in my dehydrator.

Pumpkin Seeds: I buy pumpkin seeds from *Austria's Finest*. I buy a big bag and put it in my second refrigerator. I also buy their raw pumpkin seed oil, which is just amazing. You can call (703) 360-5766 or visit their website at www.austrianpumpkinoil.com. I try to buy enough Austrian pumpkin seeds so I get free freight.

VANILLA: I also purchase vanilla in bulk from *Sun Organics.* You can place an order at www.sunorganic.com or 888-269-9888. I used to buy one bottle of vanilla at a time but I now buy four at a time. I don't save on the bottle price, but I do save on shipping and handling. It just makes sense to buy four at a time. Plus by the time I start my third bottle, it acts as a reminder to place another order. I go through a lot of vanilla right now, because I just love adding vanilla to homemade almond milk.

COCONUT BUTTER/OIL: I use coconut butter and oils when preparing food, and I also use these items on my skin. So, I get two uses out of them. Did you know coconut is good for our skin?

CHICK PEAS: This item will keep for almost forever. I always buy chick peas in bulk and have them on hand to make my own raw hummus and falafels.

DATES: The best dates come from *The Date People* in southern California. They grow a variety of dates including rare types. You can go to their webpage at www.datepeople.net and then call (760) 359-3211 to place an order. Leave a message and they will call you back. Their dates will last over a year, if you store them in a plastic freezer bag in your freezer or even in the fridge. However, when eating them right after they harvest, they are just yummy!

SEA VEGETABLES: The place to order sea vegetables is from *Rising Tide* in California. I usually buy sea palm, hizki, nori and other sea vegetables. You can visit their website at www.loveseaweed.com or call 707-964-5663. I purchase enough so I get wholesale pricing. It usually takes me three-quarters of a year to use up the items, but I get better pricing and Rising Tide's quality is impeccable. I even save on freight.

USE EVERY OUNCE...NO JOKE!

Pulp from Juicing: After I make my green juice, I save the pulp and turn it into crackers or vegetable tortillas.

Leftovers: Yes, save the leftover salads, the lettuce and veggies! I add flax meal and spices to leftover salads. Then, I mix them all together and spread on Teflex liner sheets and dehydrate. Walla, I now have crackers! No waste!

Pulp from Juicing Green Juice: Another good tip I just discovered is to dehydrate (at 105 degrees) the pulp from green juice. Spread the pulp on a Teflex sheet and place in your dehydrator. It usually takes 10 hours to dry in a dehydrator. After it is dry, I mortar and pestle it to a powder and add it to my cats' food instead of buying green powders for them. You can also save the green pulp and turn it into crackers. The green pulp is one of the ingredients used to make *Garden Veggie Crackers* (p.108).

Almonds: I do not waste a single ounce of almond. After I make almond milk, I save the pulp and turn the pulp into crackers, croutons and scones. I really *milk*, yes every pun intended, those almonds.

GROW & MAKE YOUR OWN...

JUICE YOUR OWN DRINKS: Get your juicer or Vitamix out and make your own lemonade, watermelon juice, and orange juice. Not only will you save money, but it is healthier for you. It is so refreshing, as well. Plus, the juice looks beautiful flowing out of the machine. You feel a sense of accomplishment when you pour the juice into a beautiful glass and drink up.

WATER: I have a water purification system on my kitchen sink, where it not only takes all the "ickies" out of the water, it also increases the pH. If you were to visit me at home, you will see that I fill pitchers of water every day and drink from the pitchers opposed to drinking water straight from the faucet. Plus, I refill my water bottles with the healthy water and take them with me when I leave the house. I haven't bought cases of water in eons because I keep refilling my bottles. So, I save money and I save the landfill by not filling it up with more bottles.

GROW PLANTS FROM SEEDS: Buy seeds and grow them yourself. I have found a wholesaler who sells organic seeds. I grow my own sunflower sprouts, and sprout my own lentils and mung beans. Then, of course, I can turn them into veggie burgers, salads, drinks, or whatever my heart and mind desire to create. Check out *Tiensvold Farms*, they are organic and their prices are economical. You can visit their website at www.localharvest.com or call 308-327-3135.

GROWING PLANTS YEAR-ROUND: I purchased a *three-season greenhouse* and a small *starter greenhouse*, so I can grow my own vegetables all year round and be self-sustaining. When you grow your own food, it costs you pennies and you have the fun and thrill of growing your own food. I enjoy watching the sunflower seeds I plant grow. It's fun, healthy, rewarding and economical.

OTHER WAYS TO LIVE RESOURCEFULLY

These are just a few more ways I have learned to be resourceful. As I mentioned, it's now like a game for me as I challenge myself to think of other clever and innovative ideas. While Living Dynamically, I am also Living Resourcefully, and, ironically, I have improved the quality of my life in every way and I have not taken away from it. If you have any other great ideas, please contact me at my web site at www.livingdyanmically.com and share.

REPAIR YOUR SHOES: Take your shoes to the shoe repairman. I've been doing this forever. My shoe repairman repairs my shoes until we can longer repair them.

BUY IN BULK: You can do this in so many ways. Buy toilet paper, paper towels, dish detergent, even kitty litter at a warehouse club. Not only are the larger sizes more economical, you save time and your valuable time is worth a lot! Besides, you save gas not having to run to the store every week for these items. I love just going down to my basement to get another role of paper towels or toilet paper, especially in the middle of a snow storm.

AVOID PEAK HOURS: In some parts of the country you can run your dishwasher, washer, and dryer after peak hours and weekends, and your electricity rate will be lower. Look at your utility bill and see when your peak hours are and the rate difference. It adds up.

HANG YOUR LAUNDRY: Hang your laundry instead of using the dryer. The sun and fresh air are great for your clothes and you save electricity. If you aren't allowed to hang clothes where you live, then hang as much as you can on a shower rod. You will save on utility bills, plus you also save on the wear and tear of your clothes. Dryers really wear out your clothes. Another benefit is that you will get fresh air and sunshine—good old vitamin D—you will save money at the same time.

I can't seem to hang clothes out where I live, not because I am not allowed to, because the birds always put the bulls eye on my clothes and they dive bomb them, especially after they eat my blueberries. I'm not kidding. The clothes end up dirtier than before I wash. So if your birds are better behaved than mine, please hang your clothes out. And if you have any suggestions, please send them my way.

COMPUTER USAGE: Turn your computer off when you are not using it. Don't let it run all day. You can save $100 a year doing this.

Recycle: Thank God my town recycles cans and bottles, so no longer are they going in to a landfill. Plus, some very ingenious people, including Whole Foods Market, turn their bottles into very cute tote bags. *ZakDesigns.com* whose bowls and spoons I just love, make their products out of recycled plastic. I think we should have been more ingenious years ago. But it's better late than never.

EVERY LAST OUNCE: When you get to the bottom of a tube, a bottle of cream, shampoo, or molding clay, cut the tube open; you will find you have another week or two of product depending on how you use the product.

REUSE: Besides washing out my plastic bags, I even wash out and re-use my plastic disposable cups and flatware. I'm always thinking up ways to save.

PACK A LUNCH: Packing a lunch instead of going out to a restaurant will save so much money.

RENEGOTIATE: Twice a year, give your cellphone, landline and television service companies a call. The reason for renegotiating your service twice a year is because the companies are always coming up with better and cheaper packages and, of course, they are not going to call you and tell you that. So you have to call them. If you have not combined these services, you can bundle your cable, landline, and internet into one bill, and that will save even more money.

PAY OFF CREDIT CARDS: Pay your credit card off every month, so you don't pay any interest. If you don't already have a credit card that offers incentives without paying an annual fee, transfer over to another company. I have an Amazon Visa and I get coupons every month which I use to get books, and other items, even coconut water. I just make a list of what I want and when the coupons come, I send for the items I have on my list. It's like Christmas money, but I'm not spending any money! As you know, there are all kinds of credit cards that give you coupons, such as L.L. Bean. I saved my coupons for a new winter raincoat I desperately needed. Some people have credit cards that earn them airline tickets and others earn Macy's money. Get what works for you.

BEAUTY SALON: When you get your hair cut, don't get it blow dried. You'll save money. Don't get the extra special conditioners that are supposed to make your hair last longer. They really don't. Plus, it adds cost to your bill. Extend your interval between cuts by one week.

MAGAZINES & NEWSPAPERS: Once I finish reading my entertainment magazines, I pass them on to my parents, they read them, and then give them to my Mom's hairdresser to read. When my Dad is finished with his Wall Street Journal, he passes it on to me to read. When I'm finished reading newspapers, I either recycle them or line the bottom of Tweety's cages.

RUBBERBANDS & SUCH: I save rubberbands from my mail, newspaper and vegetables. I reuse them as well. The vegetable rubberbands work well to hold the net on the jars I use for sprouting. I even save the twisties and baggies that my vegetables and wheat grass come in and reuse them. I don't have to buy rubberbands, because I collect them every day off my newspaper. I've been recycling these for years and saving money.

HOME TEMPERATURE: I save money by setting my heater in the winter at 60 degrees. If I'm chilly, I just wear a sweater. I save money and, frankly, my sinuses feel better. As long as it's not too chilly for Tweety, the rest of us (dogs, cats, and I) are okay at 60. I do the same in reverse in the summer time. Before I turn the air conditioning on in the summer time, I use the ceiling fans. It's amazing how much cooler my house stays with ceiling fans. Because of the fans, I don't have to turn the air conditioning on until it gets really hot and then I set it at 78.

VEHICLE & FUEL: I drive a Prius, so I save on gas as well. Plus, I know where the cheapest gas is and that's where I top my tank. As a sales rep, I do a lot of driving and I am all over the place so I make it a point to know where the most economical places are to buy gas and that is exactly where I buy it.

GROW YOUR OWN FOOD: I have been blessed. Every late winter a local farmer, friend who lives near me, believe it not, has come to my house and planted all my big pots with herbs and tomato plants he started in his greenhouse. Just this year, I purchased a greenhouse and I am now able to grow vegetable plants from seed. By the time spring arrives, I will have beautiful herbs and tomato plants. Spring through fall, I can walk out my kitchen door and cut whatever herbs I need for whatever I am making. Not only am I saving money, but the herbs are fresh and tasty. The tomato plants begin to produce in the summer and I enjoy watching them grow in addition to eating them. There is nothing like a fresh tomato. If you aren't as lucky as I to have a wonderful farmer close at hand, you can start your plants in your window sill whether you live in a city in an apartment or in the country. Be creative and, of course, be resourceful.

The more you can do for yourself and not rely on others, the better you will be. Besides, you'll feel more fulfilled. It's a wonderful thing. All of the things I mention may, in themselves, not sound like they would add up to much but put them all together and they make a big difference.

RESOURCEFULNESS FOR YOUR PETS

Even my pets (Taffy, Charlie, Kitty, Shorty, Tweety & Riley) have learned to be resourceful. If they can be resourceful, so can we humans! I know I could save money if I didn't have my pets, but they are my babies, so that's just not an option.

INVISIBLE FENCE: I highly recommend an Invisible Fence. It keeps everyone safe. I also have a wooden fence. It keeps us in, everyone else out, and keeps my dogs safe. It's worth it. When you have a fence up, people don't go traipsing through your property. It remains private property.

If you have dogs and you have an Invisible Fence like I do, purchase your batteries for a year and get the guarantee. Yes, it's more expensive at first, but it is actually cheaper in the long run. Your batteries are sent to you every quarter, which reminds you to change the batteries, plus you have the guarantee if anything breaks down or wears out, they replace it. This is less expensive than paying a large service call or having to buy new collars. I have three dogs, so it's definitely worth it.

BULK FOOD: I buy pet food in bulk, as well. I buy the large 40 pound bags of dry dog food. I also buy the large bags of dry cat and parrot food. Again, buying in bulk saves money, time, and gas. I used to buy canned dog food, and I now supplement the dogs' dry food with the little pouches. It's cheaper to purchase the pouches plus there are no cans to recycle. I also scout around to see which store has the cheapest food of the brands that I prefer to purchase, so I save money that way as well.

CAT LITTER: Buy kitty litter at your warehouse club in big boxes. It is so much cheaper than buying at the grocery store or at a pet store.

PET TOYS: Buy pet toys during the "After" Christmas sales. Or, see what you have that can be turned in to a toy. My parrot, Tweety, just loves the coconuts he gets each morning. Parrot toys cost $25 to $30 or more, so not only do I save on the price of the coconuts (I buy in bulk), I save money on parrot toys and Tweety is a happy camper...er...parrot. Besides giving Tweety coconuts, I also give him the empty paper towel cores, as well as the toilet paper cores. He loves to chew on them. Give your dogs and cats your old socks, tennis balls, etc. You have plenty of "stuff" around the house that can be turned in to toys without spending money.

BEVERAGES
BREAD & CRACKERS
FINGER FOODS
SALADS & SOUPS
ENTREES
DESSERTS

The recipes in this section come from
the many people who have influenced me
and touched my life
by attending the monthly Raw Potlucks
I organize in Royersford, Pennsylvania.

R
E
C
I
P
E
S

Raw beverages are a quick and easy way
to get healthy fruits and vegetables into your body.
They are much easier for your body to digest.
You don't have to chew, so for once you get to be lazy
and have a positive impact on your body.
How often does that happen?

Fresh juice and smoothies are something most everyone enjoys
and they are very simple and very easy to make.
You'll need a juicer and a blender.
The recipes in this section are a great place to begin,
if you want to transition slowly into your new lifestyle.

I begin each morning juicing and blending.
I use my Tribest Greenstar Juicer to juice wheat grass,
and then I use my Vita-Mix to prepare a fruit smoothie.
I rarely ever deviate from this morning ritual.

In fact, one of my long-time (elderly) friends had heard me rave about
the positive impact of juicing for years and she was convinced
it would be way too difficult to transition her lifestyle.
So she didn't even bother to try to juice in her kitchen.
But, after she attended a Potluck and tried the Green Smoothie,
she commented, "I can do that. It's easy!"
Today she makes her own fresh juice and smoothies.

WHEAT GRASS DRINK

LISA MONTGOMERY

I drink this every morning. When drinking wheat grass, DO NOT chug it down.
Take a mouthful and hold it in your mouth, swish it around for a few seconds before swallowing.
Drink your entire glass mouthful by mouthful. Do not drink it down quickly.

Go to www.livingdynamically.com and watch me make this drink.

Prep: 10 minutes

Wheat Grass

Take a handful of wheat grass and run it through your juicer. Beginners, juice enough so you have 1-2 ounces. I juice 5-8 ounces a day.

WHERE TO BUY WHEAT GRASS?
I buy wheat grass in flats from my local health market.
If you do not have a market near you that sells wheat grass, you can purchase it online and have it shipped directly to you. Wheat Grass Growers in Clarks Summit, Pennsylvania can provide this service. Call 570-587-5704 to order. Or find a local wheat grass grower near you.
If your store does not carry wheat grass and sprouts, ask them to call their local produce distributor and to stock it. That's what I did! Or just grow your own wheat grass.

HOW TO HARVEST WHEAT GRASS?
I take the flats home and cut the wheat grass off of the mat with a chef's knife. I originally tried cutting the wheat grass with shears and found the sharp chef's knife works better for me. I have a friend, Loreta of Loreta's Living Foods, who grows wheat grass and sprouts. She cuts the wheat grass using a straight edge razor blade. I don't dare try her technique...must be because I cannot handle the sight of my own blood and the fact my Mom wouldn't allow me to play with sharp objects when I was growing up. I'll stick with using a chef's knife!
You choose what works best for you.

HOW TO STORE WHEAT GRASS?
After I cut the wheat grass off the mat, I store it in Ziploc bags. I add a couple of paper towels in each ziplock to soak up the moisture. I keep the bags in my refrigerator. The cut grass will stay fresh for one week.

WHY SHOULD YOU CUT THE GRASS OFF THE MAT?
You want to cut the wheat grass off the mat right away! The grass will not grow longer.
Instead, it will turn yellow and rot very quickly.

LISA'S FAVORITE GREEN JUICE

LISA MONTGOMERY

This recipe is truly my all time favorite green juice recipe. It is so yummy!
It's also very easy to make.
There are many days I make this recipe
and put it in a Ball jar and pack it in my lunch box
to drink later in the day.
Be sure your lunch box is able to keep this item cool.

Prep: 10 minutes

1 cucumber

3 celery stalks

3 kale leaves

2 apples

½ lemon, juice only

Run all the ingredients, except the lemon, through a juicer. Pour into drinking glass. Squeeze the lemon half by hand or with hand juicer, then add lemon juice to mixture. Stir well. Ready to drink!

FRESH FRUIT JUICE

There is no comparison to fresh juice.
Juice your favorite fruits to make a refreshing natural drink.

You can also freeze citrus juice in jars and store in freezer for later use,
but be sure to leave room for the juice to expand as it freezes.

It's so nice to have a glass of fresh squeezed juice anytime of the year.

Prep: 10 minutes or more
Depends on quantity

Citrus Juice

oranges

mandarins

lemons

grapefuit

limes

Fresh Summer Juice

watermelon

cantaloupe

honey melon

Use a juicer to juice the fruit of your choice.

SIMPLY SPLENDID DAILY JUICE

CHRISTY PARRY, POTLUCKER

For the most benefit, drink immediately after juicing and be sure to drink slowly.
Be sure to keep the juice in your mouth for a few seconds before swallowing.

Prep: 20 minutes

½-1 cucumber

1-2 carrots

1-2 celery stalks

½ large or 1 small beet

½ lemon, juice only

1 apple, cored

1-2 large collard leaves

Cut ingredients into size and shape suitable for your jucier.

Juice the ingredients in any order.

Enjoy as is or dilute by half with filtered water.

CHOCO NANNA SMOOTHIE

LISA MONTGOMERY

I always have a bag of frozen bananas (peels removed) in my freezer
ready to go for any occasion.
This smoothie is like having a chocolate milkshake.

Prep: 10 minutes

3 frozen bananas

1 tray of ice cubes

1-2 heaping tablespoons raw cacao
   or carob powder

1 teaspoon raw honey or agave syrup

1 young Thai coconut, meat & water

In high powered blender,

toss in all ingredients and blend until creamy.

Pour into drinking glasses and enjoy.

LISA'S BREAKFAST SMOOTHIE

LISA MONTGOMERY

In the summertime, I add frozen bananas and a tray of ice cubes to this recipe.
It makes it more cooling and refreshing.
If I add frozen bananas and ice cubes in the winter, I tend to be too cold.
I know this because I have tried it.
In the wintertime, I used to make this smoothie with frozen bananas and ice cubes
and after drinking it, I would have to put on a heating pad to keep warm,
however the cooling effect in the summer is just perfect.

I like to use blueberries, raspberries and pineapple when making this recipe.

Prep: 10 minutes

3 bananas

In blender, blend all ingredients until smooth.

1 young Thai coconut, meat & water

handful of chopped fruit and/or berries

Optional:

frozen bananas

ice cubes

WHAT CAN I DO WITH THE ALMOND PULP?
I DON'T WANT TO WASTE IT!

There are so many ways to use almond pulp. I'll give you a few. However, I challenge you to use your imagination and I am sure you will create yummy treats.

Almond Flour: Dehydrate the pulp until dry. Then put in a food processor and blend until the dry chunks turn into a flour texture. Store almond flour in an airtight container. This flour can be used for making crackers. For those of you who are not totally raw, go ahead and use the almond flour and bake with it. This flour will be fresh for a month or more as long as it is not stored in a warm environment.

Pet Treats: My pets just love this tasty treat. Go ahead and sprinkle it on your dog and cat dishes. They'll just lick it up!

Don't Have Time!: Save the pulp by storing it in a plastic bag. You can store the bag in your refrigerator or freezer until ready to use. If storing in the freezer, take out the pulp and let it defrost.

Croutons: Recipe courtesy of Cherie Soria. You'll need about 2 cups of almond pulp. Croutons can be used to top your salads and soups or just eat as a snack.

FROM *THE RAW FOOD REVOLUTION DIET* BY CHERIE SORIA

Almond Pulp from Almond Milk
Prep: 10 minutes
Dehydrate: 18-24 hours

2 cups almond pulp

1 zucchini, finely diced

1 cup flax seeds, ground

2 tablespoons yeast flakes

2 teaspoons fresh Italian herbs

½ teaspoon salt

Optional:

2 teaspoons garlic, crushed

Mix all items in a bowl.
Then spread on Teflex liner sheets and cut into small cubes or spoon small portion of mixture and drop on liner sheets.
Then dehydrate until crisp; about 18-24 hours.
Store croutons in airtight container.

Almond Bread
Almond Scones
Arnold's Original Carrot Bread
Green Bread
Leftover Salad Crackers
Flax Crackers
Pumpkin Spice Beauty Snack
Sweet Pumpkin Topper Cracker
Garden Veggie Crackers
Zesty Flax Crackers

People think they have to give up bread and crackers
just because they go raw.
It just isn't so!

The variety of raw breads and crackers one can make is endless.
So not to worry,
you still have your comfort food of bread and crackers,
only now it's good for you.

BREAD & CRACKERS

Equipment that is used for dehydrated bread & crackers:
You will need a food processor, high powered blender
and dehydrator with Teflex liner trays.

Dehydrate at 105 degrees, unless otherwise specifed.

The Purpose of Soaking Nuts and Seeds:
Nuts and seeds contain a high amount of enzyme inhibitors
which prevent the nuts from sprouting prematurely
and this can strain your digestive system.
When you soak nuts, it neutralizes the enzyme inhibitors
and helps to encourage the production of beneficial enzymes.
In turn, the enzymes increase the nutrition (add more vitamins)
of nuts and seeds and make them easier to digest.

How to Soak Nuts and Seeds:
I prefer to soak/sprout nuts in the morning
before I head out the door for work
or in the evening, so they soak overnight.
In any case, the nuts will have been soaking in water
for at least 8 hours.
So soak your nuts when it is most convenient for you.

ALMOND BREAD

CHERIE SORIA, LIVING LIGHT CULINARY ARTS INSTITUTE
FORT BRAGG, CALIFORNIA

This bread is delicious. It is best when served right out of the dehydrator.
Yum, fresh, warm bread! Or if you like, make scones.

Be sure to save enough pulp from your almond milk for this recipe.

Prep: 10 minutes
Dehydrate: 6-8 hours at 105 degrees

6 cups almond pulp (from almond milk)
1¼ cups flax meal
½ cup flax oil
½ cup olive oil
1 teaspoon sea salt

Place all ingredients in a large bowl and mix well. Place a portion of the batter between two non-stick dehydrator sheets, then use a rolling pin to spread the batter until it is about ¼ inch thick. Cut into slices and place on a dehydrator tray using a spatula. Dehydrate at 105 degrees for 6 to 8 hours. Bread should be firm and moist. If stored in an airtight container, it will last up to 4 days and up to 2 months in the freezer.

How about Almond Scones?

CHERIE SORIA, LIVING LIGHT CULINARY ARTS INSTITUTE

6 cups almond pulp (from almond milk)
1¼ cups flax meal
½ cup flax oil
½ cup olive oil
½ teaspoon sea salt
1 teaspoon cinnamon
optional:
1 cup raisins or dried cranberries
½ cup pitted, chopped dates

Place all ingredients in a large bowl and mix well. Stir in optional ingredients.
Form the dough into a round shape about 1 inch thick.
Cut into wedges and dehydrate for 6 hours. Serve warm.

ARNOLD'S ORIGINAL CARROT BREAD

MICHELLE SCHULMAN, RAW CHEF; ARNOLD'S WAY, LANDSDALE, PENNSYLVANIA

Michelle is on her own amazing raw, healing journey as you know from reading her story in this book. In fact, she is working on her very own raw cookbook, which will be coming out in the future. Michelle is a raw chef at Arnold's Way, a raw restaurant in Lansdale, Pennsylvania. She is also an opera singer, so if you take one of her cooking classes or if she caters for you, you can bet she will also sing for you...mmm...maybe that's where the term "singing for your supper" came from.

Hint: To speed up the process, use shredded carrots instead of carrot pulp from juicing.

Soak Flax & Buckwheat: Overnight
Prep: 15 minutes
Dehydrate: 1-2 days

STEP 1 - SOAKING INSTRUCTIONS

To create 3 cups of soaked flax/buckwheat:

1 cup flax dry

1 cup buckwheat dry

(Replace buckwheat with quinoa, sesame or sunflower seeds)

Add enough water so that they are covered by 1 inch in a large bowl. Use filtered water. Let sit 1 hour on the countertop and stir occasionally. Make sure all seeds are moist but not over soaked. Adjust the amount of water if necessary, or strain if the seeds are too wet. Cover and refrigerate overnight. You should have 3 cups to make the bread recipes.

STEP 2

makes 3 dehydrator trays of living bread

3 cups soaked flax and buckwheat

3 cups carrot pulp

6 ounces (or less) olive oil

2 level tablespoons celtic rock salt

(use less if using Himalayan fine ground sea salt)

Use a large capacity food processor with S blade to process all ingredients for several minutes. Be sure to process until flax has cracked and opened. The mixture will continue to come together. On a Teflex sheet, spread ⅓ of the mix, spreading evenly, and leaving 1½ inches from the edge of all sides of the Teflex. Score into triangles or squares, if desired, with the end of a spatula. Dry overnight at 105 degrees.

Continue with STEP 3 on next page...

GREEN BREAD

MICHELLE SCHULMAN, RAW CHEF; ARNOLD'S WAY, LANDSDALE, PENNSYLVANIA

This is one of many variations for making Green Bread.
Follow the same directions for the Carrot Bread. The only difference is the ingredients.

Soak Flax & Buckwheat: Overnight
Prep: 15 minutes
Dehydrate: 1-2 days

3 cups soaked flax and buckwheat

2 cups baby spinach leaves
(or any greens)

1 cup carrot pulp

Garlic/onion mixture to taste
(garlic, onion, water in Vita-mix)

6 ounces olive oil

1 level tablespoon Celtic Sea Salt

Follow STEP 1 & directions for STEP 2 on page 102, but use ingredients listed on this page for STEP 2.

Do not begin Step 3 until mixture has been dehydrated for at least 8 hours.

STEP 3

The next morning, flip the bread by using another dehydrator tray on top. Remove the top tray and peel the Teflex off the back of the bread. Place bread back in the dehydrator for another day and the bread will be done in the morning. If you check sooner, and it is dry, enjoy! Bread that is fully dried lasts at least 10 to 12 months in a Tupperware container. Bread that is NOT fully dried will go floppy when stored and does not have a long shelf life. This is yummy, but should be eaten right away! If you find your bread is floppy and you want to harden it, just place it in the dehydrator to complete drying!

To clean the Teflex trays, put them in soapy water for 30 minutes to easily clean off.

If you want to make enough flax/buckwheat mix to make bread again 2 days after this batch is done, soak a lot. Soaked flax/buckwheat will last in the refrigerator for 3 to 4 days. It may sprout (you'll see tails begin to grow), but that's okay.

LEFT OVER SALAD CRACKERS

LISA MONTGOMERY

You will notice there are no specific quantities for this recipe.

Soak Nuts: 8 hours
Soak Flax Seeds: 2-4 hours
Dehydrate: Overnight or until desired dryness

nuts
flax seeds
leftover salad

Soak nuts and flax seeds in clean, pure water.

Drain and rinse the nuts and flax seeds.

In a food processor, add all the ingredients and blend until the mixture has a dough-like consistency.

You may need to add water to get the dough consistency.

Spread the mixture on Teflex sheets, score and dehydrate.

Half way through the drying process, remove crackers from the Teflex sheets and turn them over.

Continue dehydrating until dried to desired consistency.

FLAX CRACKERS

LORRAINE GODSOE, POTLUCKER

This was a hit at one of my Potlucks. The pate will keep in the refrigerator for about two weeks, that is unless you eat it before the two weeks are up.

Prep Crackers: 20 minutes
Cracker Mix Sits: 24 hours
Soak Sunflower seeds: 6-8 hours
Dehydrate: 18-24 hours

4 cups flaxseed (brown or golden)

1 cup sunflower seeds (without shell)

2 large onions

6 stalks celery

2-3 carrots

1 red pepper

½ cup sundried tomatoes in herbs and oil

8 medium garlic cloves

1 bunch parsley or cilantro

1 tablespoon Celtic sea salt

2 teaspoons coriander

Braggs to taste (optional)

2 cups water

Partially grind flaxseed in blender and place in a large bowl. Set aside.

Soak sunflower seeds for 6-8 hours in water. (You will use these on day two.)

Cut the vegetables into large chunks and blend in blender along with remainder of ingredients. Pour blended mixture in large bowl and mix thoroughly with flaxseeds. Cover with a platter and let stand at room temperature for about 24 hours.

Don't forget to drain sunflower seeds after 6-8 hours of soaking. After dough has sat for 24 hours, stir in sunflower seeds.

Spread mixture on Teflex sheets or parchment paper, score and dehydrate for 12 hours. Flip and continue dehydrating for another 12 hours. They are done when dry and crisp.

They can be stored in plastic bags in freezer.

Makes about 7½ dehydrator trays.

The mixture can be frozen and used at a later time.

PUMPKIN SPICE BEAUTY SNACK

JANICE INNELLA, THE BEAUTY CHEF, POTLUCKER

This recipe is my favorite for spicy crackers. I make it often.
Everyone I serve it to just loves it.

I use Austria's Finest pumpkin seeds. They are superior!

Soak Pumpkin Seeds: 8 hours
Sprout Pumpkin Seeds: 4 hours or less
Soak Flax Seeds: 4 hours
Prep: 70 minutes (includes waiting time)
Dehydrate: 18 hours at 115 degrees

2 cups pumpkin seeds, soaked & sprouted

1 cup golden flaxseed, soaked in 2 cups water

1 cup pumpkin seeds, ground

1 cup golden flaxseed, ground

2 cups pure water

2 lemons, juiced

2 tablespoons lemon zest

1 teaspoon cayenne pepper

1 tablespoon Celtic sea salt or ½ tablespoon Himalayan pink sea salt

4 tablespoons olive oil, hemp seed oil or Austrian pumpkin seed oil

1 large red onion, minced finely

1 tablespoon Caraway seed, ground on side

Soak pumpkin seeds for 8 hours, then rinse and sprout for 4 hours. Soak flax seeds in 2 cups of water and let sit for 4 hours. In a large bowl, mix by hand all ingredients thoroughly. Let sit for 20 minutes. Then use a spatula to evenly spread mixture onto about 5 Teflex sheets. Score into small 1 inch crackers or larger. Set dehydrator to 115 degrees and dry for 12 hours. Flip trays with another tray on top, then peel off Teflex sheet and dehydrate for another 6 hours. Store in cool dry container.

Beauty Note: This recipe is a low carb, low calorie snack especially good for those with Diabetes. Beautifying effects are the rich omegas in the pumpkin seeds and the high fiber in the flax seed. Beauty from the inside out.

SWEET PUMPKIN TOPPER CRACKER

JANICE INNELLA, THE BEAUTY CHEF, POTLUCKER

As spicy as the Pumpkin Spice Beauty Snack is, this sweet pumpkin recipe is sweet.
The two are a fabulous combo to serve together.

Soak Pumpkin Seeds: 8 hours
Sprout Pumpkin Seeds: 4 hours
Soak Flax Seeds: 4 hours
Soak Dried Cranberries: Until soft
Soak Dry Coconut: In 1 cup of water until soft
Dehydrate: 24-26 hours at 115 degrees

2 cups pumpkin seeds, soaked & sprouted

1 cup golden flaxseed soaked in 2 cups water

1 cup pumpkin seeds, ground

4 Gala apples, minced in food processor

2 tablespoons cinnamon

1 teaspoon nutmeg

1 teaspoon cardamom seed, ground or powdered

2 tablespoons vanilla extract (non-alcohol) or 2 raw beans split and scraped

½ teaspoon clove

½ teaspoon allspice or garam masala

4 tablespoons coconut butter

4 tablespoons pumpkin seed oil

½ cup agave syrup

2 limes, juiced

1 teaspoon Celtic sea salt

1 cup dried cranberries, unsweetened & soaked

1 cup dry coconut, soaked

Soak pumpkin seeds for 8 hours then rinse and then sprout for 4 hours. Soak flax seeds in 2 cups of water and let sit for 4 hours. Soak cranberries and coconut until soft.

In a large bowl, add everything except cranberries and coconut. Mix thoroughly by hand. In food processor using S blade, pulse and blend cranberries and coconut. Add to mixture and stir until well blended. Spread mixture on Teflex sheets and dehydrate for 12 hours at 115 degrees, then turn over and dehydrate for another 12-16 hours. Texture should be chewy with a little crunch. Makes about 5 trays. Store in cool, dry containers for up to 3 months.

GARDEN VEGGIE CRACKERS

RAW CHEF DAN, QUINTESSENCE, MANHATTAN

For a variety of flavors of this cracker, try adding dried coconut, chili powder
or for a buttery flavor, add pine nuts.

Save: Green Juice Pulp
Prep: 10 minutes
Dehydrate: 8 hours at 95 degrees

2 cups mixed pulp (from green juices)

½ cup flax seeds (grind to powder and add ⅔ cup water)

½ cup flax seeds, whole

1 teaspoon sea salt

1 teaspoon agave (optional)

In a large bowl, mix all ingredients together thoroughly.

Then spread mixture on Teflex dehydrator sheet so it is ¼ inch thick.

Place in dehydrator and dry at 95 degrees for 4 hours.

Then flip over the mixture and dehydrate for another 4 hours.

Be sure to remove the Teflex sheet at this time.

After 8 hours, it should be dry, but still have some flexibility.

Cut into desired shapes.

ZESTY FLAX CRACKERS

JOEL ODHNER, PERSONAL CHEF & NUTRITION COACH

PREP: 20 MINUTES
DEHYDRATE: 8-10 HOURS

6 cups flax, ground

3 cups flax, whole

¾ bunch celery

2 carrots

½ red onion, chopped

½ cup sundried tomato

4 garlic cloves

cayenne pepper to taste

½ cup fresh or ¼ cup dry herbs of your choice

Grind flax.

Then add both the ground and whole flax together and set aside.

Combine remaining ingredients in blender.

Cover with water.

Blend well.

Mix blended mixture with flax.

Spread on Teflex sheets.

Cut into size cracker of choice.

Dehydrate for 8 to 10 hours.

Kale Chips
Basic Nut Creamy Cheese/Moc Cream Cheese
Chedder Cheeze (Red Pepper Cheese)
Red Bell Pepper Cheese
Cheddar Nut Cheesy Dip (with a little kick)
Marinated Mushrooms
Guacamole Stuffed Mushrooms
Onion Dip
Turkish Sundried Tomato Pate
Pumpkinseed Pate
Hummus
SunFlower Pate
Green Fried Tomatoes
Sweet Cinnamon Mixed Nuts
Spicy Hot Nuts
Trail Mix
Pix Up Stix Veggies

Foods I can eat with my hands are my favorite.
I have been known to have meals of just finger foods and appetizers.
Let's face it, isn't it more fun to try a buffet of tasty foods
then just a regular every day sit down meal?

The recipes in this section are a simple way to get people to try raw food.
For example, if you take a raw hummus (most people eat hummus)
or a dip to a family or friend gathering, you will notice that your treat may be
devoured and all you'll have to take home is your empty serving dish.
Besides, the recipes are easy to make.
You don't have to be a brain surgeon—no offense to the brain surgeons—
to make a salsa, hummus or dip.
They are quick, simple and tasty!

Try adding some of the dip and pate recipes to greens and have a meal.

FINGER FOODS

KALE CHIPS

Lisa Montgomery

Who needs standard American potato chips?
You won't ever miss them once you start eating kale chips.
It's also a healthy way to get more greens in your beautiful body.
So when you feel the need to munch on something or when your emotional stuff is kicking up,
pull out a bag of kale chips.
You can even eat a whole bag and not have to worry about weight gain
and overeating something unhealthy.

Prep: 5 minutes
Dehydrate: 4-8 hours/overnight at 105 degrees

kale, shredded
sea salt
pumpkin seed oil

Remove the stems from the kale, then shred the leaves. Toss the kale in a little sea salt and pumpkin seed oil and mix all together, then place the shredded kale on Teflex liner sheets and dehydrate overnight. When I wake up in the morning, the kale chips are ready to munch on. Bag the kale chips in a plastic baggy.

Try marinating the kale in a raw barbeque sauce or raw cheese sauce. They are so amazing.

Basic Nut Creamy Cheese/Moc Cream Cheese

Raw Chef Dan, Quintessence, Manhattan

I do so many things with this recipe.
I use it as a dressing, in a nori roll, as a topping on pizza and a dip for kale chips.
It is so versatile. I also love to add dill, chives, scallions, and other items.
So, use your creativity.

Prep: 5 minutes

½ cup pine nuts or really raw cashews
½ cup macadamia nuts
1 cup water
¼ cup lemon juice
½ teaspoon sea salt

Blend all ingredients until creamy and smooth. Add enough water to blend.

CHEDDER CHEEZE (RED PEPPER CHEESE)

MICHELLE SCHULMAN, RAW CHEF, ARNOLD'S WAY, LANDSDALE, PENNSLVANIA

I use this as a cheese on crackers, in lasagna and even on greens.
Honestly, I put it on almost everything!
Chedder Cheeze lasts up to 10 days in the refrigerator.
It is particularly good slathered on Arnold's Carrot Bread *(p.102)* with veggies over it.
A very hardy meal! Also yummy in celery sticks as a crunchy snack!

This recipe makes about 6½ cups, so you may want to cut the recipe in half
or just store in the fridge and use as often as you like until it's gone!

Prep: 10 minutes

2½-3 cups red pepper spears

1 cup soaked almonds

3 cups cashews

2 tablespoons Celtic salt

1-3 teaspoons agave syrup, to taste

4 ounces lemon juice

Filtered water- *just enough
to make it blend into a "pate"*

In the food processor with an S blade, add all the ingredients except filtered water.

Process the mixture until it doesn't move anymore. Then, begin to add small amounts of filtered water to the desired consistency.

Adjust the seasoning, if desired. Add lemon and salt if bland. Add Agave if the mixture is too salty.

RED BELL PEPPER CHEESE

RAW CHEF DAN, QUINTESSENCE, MANHATTAN

Soak Chipotle Pepper: Until rehydrated
Prep: 10-15 minutes

1 medium red bell pepper
½ teaspoon sea salt
½ chipotle pepper, soaked
2 tablespoons lemon juice

Blend ingredients in a blender until smooth.
Then add the nuts.

½ cup macadamia nuts
½ cup pine nuts

Blend nuts until creamy.
Add water if necessary.

CHEDDAR NUT CHEESY DIP (WITH A LITTLE KICK)

JANICE INNELLA, THE BEAUTY CHEF, POTLUCKER

This is another recipe I use in a variety of ways.
It's great as a cheese on crackers, in lasagna, and on greens. Yum, yum, yum!

You can dehydrate this cheese mixture in your dehydrator and it will become a hard cheese.
Then, grate it as you would traditional cheese and toss it on salads.

Soak Cashews: 30 minutes
Soak Sundried Tomatoes: Until rehydrated
Prep: 10 minutes

2 cups cashews, soaked

½-1 red pepper

⅓ red onion

1 lemon (juice only)

4 tablespoons raw olive oil

1 teaspoon chipotle chili (dry)

3 sundried tomatoes, soaked

1 garlic clove (for extra kick)

1½ teaspoons Celtic sea salt

½ cup pure water.

Place all ingredients in a high powered blender and blend until creamy smooth.

Use as spread or dip.
You can even use as a salad dressing.

HOW ABOUT HARD CHEESE?

To create a hard cheese,
dehydrate mixture at 105 degrees for 24 hours.

MARINATED MUSHROOMS

LISA MONTGOMERY

Marinated mushrooms are yummy and I love to have these in my fridge.
They are very easy to prepare. I eat them as a side dish and put them on salads.

I bought a marinator from Tupperware and it is perfect
for storing and marinating mushrooms.

Soak Nuts: 8 hours
Dehydrate: Overnight or until desired dryness

mushrooms, any variety

tamari, wheat free

raw pumpkin seed oil

agave syrup

1-2 garlic cloves, finely minced

red onion, finely chopped

oregano or rosemary,
fresh & finely chopped

Wash the mushrooms and set aside.

Mix the remaining ingredients together.

Do a taste test, to get the desired flavor.

Add the mushrooms to the mixture and toss.

Be sure to cover all mushrooms with marinade mixture.

Store in an airtight container in fridge and use within week.

GUACAMOLE STUFFED MUSHROOMS

PEGGY O'NEILL, POTLUCKER

Prep: 20 minutes

40 button mushrooms

2 avocados

1 small tomato

1 Chile pepper

¼ sweet onion

salt & pepper, to taste

Optional:
paprika and olive slices

Clean mushrooms and remove the stems.
In a food processor, blend avocados, tomato, Chile pepper and onion until smooth.
Then fill the center of the mushrooms with the mixture.
Garnish the top with a sprinkle of paprika and/or olive slices.

Variation: Toss the mushrooms with balsamic vinegar and let them marinate in the refrigerator for several hours before stuffing.

ONION DIP

ANONYMOUS POTLUCKER

Be sure to add in the onions by hand, after blending the nuts and water.
For variety, try adding diced scallions.

Prep: 10 minutes
Chill: 1-2 hours before serving

2 cups macadamia nuts

¾-1 cup water

1 teaspoon sea salt

1 cup onions, diced

In a blender or food processor, blend macadamia nuts, water, and sea salt until smooth and creamy.

Start with ¾ cup water and add more only if needed to make mixture blend.

Keep this as thick as you can and make sure it's as smooth and creamy as possible when done.

Remove from machine and add in the onions by hand. Mix gently and chill.

TURKISH SUNDRIED TOMATO PATE

JANICE INNELLA, THE BEAUTY CHEF, POTLUCKER

This is another one of my all-time favorite pates. It has a bit of kick and zing.
Your taste buds will definitely not get bored when you eat this.
It's great on salads and crackers.
I like to add a slice of tomato and avocado on a cracker and top with an olive.

Cut off the hard tips of the figs and be sure to not throw out the water from soaked figs.

Soak Sundried Tomatoes: Until rehydrated
Soak Figs: Until soft
Prep: 20 minutes
Dehydrate: 12-24 hours

2 cups sundried tomatoes, soaked

1 cup black mission figs, soaked

1 red chili

1 Sarrano chili

1 jalapeno

1 teaspoon chipotle chili

1 teaspoon agave nectar or raw honey

1 garlic clove

1 tablespoon pumpkinseed oil

1 tablespoon raw olive oil

1 teaspoon cumin

1 teaspoon ground fresh coriander

1 teaspoon carraway seed, ground fresh

Soak the tomatoes and figs in separate bowls. Add just enough water to cover the figs.
Chop the chilies while tomatoes and figs are soaking.

After soaking the sundried tomatoes, press out the extra water.
Remove figs from water and save the water.

Combine all ingredients, except date water, in food processor.
Begin by pulsing, so all ingredients are blended.
Add date water a bit at a time until texture is smooth and creamy like a pate.

PUMPKINSEED PATE

JANICE INNELLA, THE BEAUTY CHEF, POTLUCKER

This is one of my all-time favorite pates.
If you prefer your pate to be chunky, then do not process as long.

Soak Pumpkin Seeds: 6 hours
Sprout Pumpkin Seeds: 4 hours
Prep Turkish Sundried Tomato Pate (p.117): 20 minutes
Prep: 15 minutes

1½ cup pumpkin seeds (Austria's Finest)

1 bunch chives

1 garlic clove

1 teaspoon Chipotle chili

1 teaspoon agave syrup

1 tablespoon Turkish Sundried Tomato Pate (p.117)

2 tablespoons pumpkin seed oil

1 bunch lavender mint (can substitute parsley)

1 teaspoon Celtic sea salt

Combine the above ingredients in food processor and blend until smooth and creamy.

HUMMUS

JOEL ODHNER, PERSONAL CHEF & NUTRITION COACH

Joel's recipe for hummus is one of my all-time favorite hummus recipes.
Anyone who tries this recipe concurs.

Soak & Sprout Garbanzo Beans: 2-3 days
Prep: 15 minutes
Chill: 1-2 hours before serving

1½ cups olive oil

3½ cups garbanzo beans, sprouted

Chill and enjoy!

1 teaspoon salt or to taste

1 cup of Veggie Mix
(chopped celery, parsley, carrots)

5 garlic cloves

Blend all ingredients in food processor.

½ cup lemon juice

SUNFLOWER PATE

NOMI SHANNON, From *THE RAW GOURMET*

Soak Sunflower Seeds: 8-12 hours
Sprout Sunflower Seeds: 4 hours
Prep: 15 minutes

2 cups sunflower seeds, soaked & sprouted

6 large carrots, cut in small pieces

1 cup lemon juice

¼ cup liquid amino (Braggs)

¼-½ cup raw tahini

½ cup chopped scallions

2-4 slices red onion, chopped in chunks

4-6 tablespoons chopped parsley

2-3 garlic cloves

½ teaspoon cayenne pepper

1 teaspoon cumin

ginger, small piece finely chopped (optional)

Place all ingredients in a food processor
and run until well blended.

GREEN FRIED TOMATOES

LISA MONTGOMERY

One of the dishes I missed when I switched to raw was green fried tomatoes.
I am now thrilled after being raw for many years,
I have finally figured out how to come up with a raw alternative.
I must confess they are so good that I rarely can wait until they are finished.

Green fried...ok so they're not fried.
These tomatoes make a great side dish to any meal.
Or just toss them on your salad.

If you dehydrate them for two days, they can be stored in an airtight container
and eaten as a snack whenever you have the urge to munch.

Use your favorite herbs.
The following go well with this dish: basil, oregano, pizza seasoning, Italian seasoning, garlic
powder, onion powder, Herbamare or a combination.

Prep: 15 minutes
Dehydrate: 4 hours to 2 days

tomatoes *(They don't have to be green.)*

olive oil

yeast flakes

Italian seasoning (herbs) and/or pizza seasoning

garlic powder

onion powder

Herbamare (salt substitute)

Thinly slice your favorite tomatoes.

Pour some olive oil in a small bowl.

On a plate combine yeast flakes, herbs and seasonings.

Then dip one tomato slice at a time in the oil and then into the herb mixture, so it is coated.

Place the coated tomato slice on a Teflex sheet and dehydrate.

After 4 to 8 hours, turn the tomatoes over until desired consistency.

Remove the Teflex sheet and continue dehydrating.

DON'T LIKE TOMATOES, HOW ABOUT STRING BEANS?
Use string beans instead of tomatoes. Or prepare both at the same time.

SWEET CINNAMON MIXED NUTS

JEAN TURNER, POTLUCKER

These were the hit at a potluck when Jean brought these scrumptious nuts.
They just blew everyone away. So easy to make! Use nuts of your choice.

Soak Nuts: Overnight
Prep: 5 minutes
Dehydrate: 24 hours at 115 degrees
Prep: 5 minutes
Dehydrate: 12 hours at 115 degrees

nuts, your choice

agave syrup

cinnamon

sea salt

Soak nuts overnight then rinse.
Spread nuts on a Teflex sheet and
dehydrate at 115 degress for 24 hours or until dry.

Place nuts in a bowl.
Coat with agave syrup and cinnamon.
Spread nuts back on Teflex sheet and sprinkle with sea salt
and dehydrate for 12 hours or until sticky.

For more sweetness, add more agave.
If you prefer salty, add more salt.

SPICY HOT NUTS

JEAN TURNER, POTLUCKER

nuts, your choice

scotch bonnet pepper *or*
 1 teaspoon cayenne pepper

cayenne pepper

agave syrup

sea salt

Chop the pepper and place in bowl of water.
If using cayenne pepper add 1 teaspoon to the water.

Then add the nuts and soak in the pepper water overnight.

Rinse the nuts and then spread them on a Teflex sheet and
dehydrate at 115 degrees for 24 hours or until dry.

Place the nuts in a bowl and coat with a little agave syrup.
Sprinkle cayenne pepper if you want the nuts to be hot.

Spread the nuts back on the Teflex sheet and sprinkle with sea
salt. Dehydrate for 12 hours.

TRAIL MIX

Bryan Taylor, Potlucker

Having trail mix available to munch on is essential,
especially for those moments when you want a quick snack or need something for a road trip.

You can also store your homemade trail mix in sealed containers and it will stay fresh for weeks!

Try making your own variation of trail mix.

Soak Almonds: Overnight
Dehydrate Almonds: 8 hours at 105 degrees
Prep: 10 minutes

2 pounds raisins

1 pound dried sweet cranberries

1¼ pounds dried pineapple (low sugar/no sugar, no sulfur)

½ pound raw almonds, whole

½ pound raw sunflower seeds

½ pound raw pumpkin seeds

All nuts and seeds are shelled.

Pineapple is cut into small pieces; about the size of a raisin.

Put all ingredients into a bowl and mix thoroughly.

PIX UP STIX VEGGIES

GARY N. GUTTMAN, POTUCKER

This is Gary's dream dish. It was his vision!
You will notice often with raw recipes that the chefs don't provide quantities.
Preparing raw food is very freeing.
Just go with your creativity and the dish always comes out wonderful.

Prep: 45 minutes

red, green & yellow peppers

celery

parsnips

carrots

asparagus

green string beans

anise

baby spinach

Italian long green peppers

Clean, cut and display veggies on a beautiful dish.

VEGGIE DIP

ground mustard

black pepper

lemon juice

garlic

apple cider vinegar

raw olive oil

In a small or medium bowl, blend dip ingredients together until you are satisfied with taste.
Put dip in a small bowl and serve with veggies.

You'll notice some recipes will not have quantities listed,
that's because your taste buds will be the judge.
Be prepared to do a bit of taste testing
as you create these delicious recipes.

Your personal preference also matters,
so use the greens, veggies, and fruits you enjoy.

This section also includes some dressings.
Have fun as you create tasty salads and soups.

COLORFUL & FESTIVE GARDEN SALAD

ESTHER MARIANO, POTLUCKER

This salad is very colorful and tasty and is a meal by itself.
It doesn't need anything else, except you and your fork.

Run a fork down the sides of the unpeeled cucumber
to make a design before slicing into thin slices.

Prep: 20 minutes

Clean and tear the following ingredients and place in a bowl:

raw spinach
Romaine & Arugula lettuce

Slice the following and add to bowl of lettuce:

1 tomato
1 onion (red or Spanish)
½ cup mushrooms
1 pepper (red, yellow, orange...your choice)
1 unpeeled cucumber

DRESSING
Drizzle a little raw virgin olive oil, raw apple cider or balsamic vinegar
or squeeze a little lemon juice on the salad to taste.
Toss and mix.

OPTIONAL TOPPINGS:
You can also add raw nuts or seeds: almonds, flax, and sesame.
Olives are also great on this salad.

CHOPPED ASIAN BEAUTY SALAD

JANICE INELLA, THE BEAUTY CHEF, POTLUCKER

Janice's recipes are always light, creative, refreshing, healthy and tasty.
Usually, her salads are beautifully layered.

Prep: 30 minutes

1 head Napa cabbage

1 bunch cilantro

1 shallot

2 Asian or Boss pears

2 red bell peppers or long hot peppers

2 red chilies

1 mango

1 pomegranate, seeds

1 cup sprouted quinoa

1 jalapeno

½ cup pumpkin seeds, ground

½ cup dry coconut flakes

1 cup bean sprouts

4 scallions

2 heads baby bok choy, hand chop

1 teaspoon cardamom

1½ tablespoons Celtic Sea Salt

1 lime

1 star fruit for garnish

In a food processor, chop the following: Napa cabbage, cilantro, shallot, pears, red peppers.

Hand chop chilies and mango.
Remove seeds from pomegranate.

In a large serving bowl add all ingredients by layering one at a time beginning with the Napa cabagge.
Sprinkle cardamom, salt and lime juice over top layer.

DRESSING

2 limes, juice

1 cup almond butter

½ cup pure water

1 teaspoon red chili paste

1 tablespoon agave nectar

1 shallot

1 tablespoon lemon grass

1 tablespoon sesame oil

1 tablespoon umeboshi plum paste

Juice the limes and add the juice to a blender. Then add all the other ingredients and blend until smooth. Pour over salad, then mix and toss.

CHOPPED BEAUTY SALAD

JANICE INNELLA, THE BEAUTY CHEF, POTLUCKER

This salad is yummy. I love topping it with ground pumpkin seeds.
You can use a food processor to chop the cabbage and kale.

Prep: 30 minutes
Chill: 1 hour

½ head red cabbage, chopped

2 red peppers, seeded & chopped

2 Gala apples, chopped

1 pound organic frozen corn
   or 4 ears of fresh corn

1 bunch of kale, leaves stripped off stem

1 pomegranate, seeds only (seasonal)

1 cup cranberries, dried or fresh

1 avocado, diced

GARNISH WITH:
pomegranate seeds
ground up pumpkin seeds.

Chop the items into small pieces and place in a large bowl. Then add the dressing ingredients and mix well.

DRESSING

1½ cups white grapefruit juice
   or white grape juice
½ tablespoon Himalayan salt or Celtic salt
Juice of one lemon

Toss the dressing ingredients with the chopped items.
Chill for 1 hour.
Before serving, mix again to allow the entire salad to marinate.

EGGPLANT & AVOCADO SALAD

ANONYMOUS POTLUCKER

Prep: 20 minutes
Marinate: 15 minutes

1 large eggplant
3 lemons, juice

4 tablespoons extra raw virgin olive oil
2 garlic cloves, chopped finely
dulse flakes and pepper to taste

2 or 3 avocados, ripe but firm
½ red onion, chopped finely

2 teaspoons raw honey

Pare and dice eggplant.
Place diced eggplant in a deep bowl and immediately cover with cold water acidulated with juice of one lemon.
Set aside.

Whisk together oil, garlic, dulse flakes, pepper and juice of one lemon.
Set aside this will be used as the dressing.

Peel and dice the avocados.
Place in bowl and toss immediately with juice of one lemon.

Drain eggplant and combine with avocados.
Add chopped onion.

Whisk dressing again and add to mixture.
Toss gently.
Set aside for about 15 minutes.
Chill if desired.
Before serving, toss gently again and drizzle with honey.

GARY'S FAMOUS CARIBBEAN SPRING SALAD

GARY N. GUTTMAN, POTLUCKER

Now you get to have fun and make this salad one of your specialties.
You will notice there are no limits to this creation.
If you love mangoes more than oranges, then add more mangoes.
The combination of all the veggies and fruit in this recipe is absolutely delicious.
Go ahead and make your version!

Prep: 10 minutes

romaine lettuce

spring mix salad

mangoes

blood oranges

naval oranges

grapefruit

pineapples

papaya

red and green grapes

radish sprouts

grape tomatoes

cucumbers

Chop the above items for a salad.
After preparing the above, combine in a bowl and toss with dressing.

Red & Green Pepper/Mango Dressing

mangoes, peeled & seed removed

lemon juice

olive oil

red & green peppers

caribbean seasoning

In a blender combine all salad dressing ingredients and blend until smooth.
Toss dressing on salad and serve.

HEMP KALE SALAD

Joel Odhner, Personal Chef & Nutrition Coach

Just like your little black dress, the basic kale salad is so versatile.
You can add whatever you want: olives, sundried tomatoes and cherry tomatoes.
Go ahead and add other items, such as avocado, peppers or your favorite veggies.

This is not a tossed salad.
The secret is to massage the kale allowing the olive oil, lemon, and salt to infuse,
thus giving it taste and texture.

This salad is great immediately after preparing, but even better over the next several days!

Prep: 15-20 minutes

2 heads kale

¼ cup extra virgin olive oil

¼ cup lemon juice

1 tablespoon sea salt

¼ cup hemp seeds

1 red bell pepper, diced

Wash kale and remove stems before chopping or shredding.

Place kale leaves in a large bowl.

Massage the kale with olive oil, lemon juice and salt.

After the kale is fully massaged, add in hemp seeds and red pepper.

LORETA'S PEAS, BEANS & LENTIL SALAD

LORETA VAINIUS, LORETA'S LIVING FOODS, MALVERN, PENNSYLVANIA

If you are lucky to live in the Malvern, Pennsylvania area,
and you are a raw foodist, then you most definitely heard about Loreta Vainius.
Loreta grows wheat grass and assorted sprouts, and sells them weekly from her home.
She also holds classes on sprouting as well.
Loreta is one who has been very instrumental in my foundational learning of raw foods.
Thank you, Loreta.

Soak Peas, Beans & Lentils: 12 hours
Sprout Peas, Beans & Lentils: 5 days
Prep: 20 minutes

Soak 3 tablespoons each peas, beans and lentils for 12 hours.

Then sprout for 5 days.

After sprouting peas, beans and lentils, place them in a bowl.

Then add the following with the sprouts:

¼ red pepper, finely chopped

Sprinkle the following over the sprouts and pepper, then toss well.

1 lemon, juice

3 tablespoons olive oil

1 teaspoon sea salt (or to taste)

1 teaspoon fresh garlic, finely minced

2-3 tablespoons fresh parsley, finely chopped

1-3 tablespoons dill, finely chopped

2 stalks celery, finely chopped

"SEAFOOD SALAD"

ANONYMOUS POTLUCKER

If you use dry sea vegetables, you will need to soak them in water until they are rehydrated. Otherwise, use a package of sea vegetable salad mix.

Soak Sea Vegetables: Until rehydrated
Prep: 20-30 minutes
Chill or Set: 30 minutes

1 package sea vegetable salad mix
  or 1 cup mixed dry sea vegetables soaked in water until rehydrated

1 cup celery, thinly sliced

1 cup carrot, shredded

½ cup fresh parsley, chopped

½ cup snipped dulse leaf

¼ cup diced onion

In a mixing bowl, combine all the ingredients.
Set aside while you prepare the dressing.

DRESSING

½ cup pine nuts
½ garlic clove
½ teaspoon kelp powder
½ teaspoon ground mustard seed
¼ teaspoon ground tumeric
⅛ teaspoon cayenne
⅓ cup water
1 teaspoon fresh lemon juice, optional
½ teaspoon Braggs Liquid Aminos or nama shoyu (or wheat free tamari)
4 drops liquid stevia extract

In a blender, combine the dressing ingredients.
Blend well and season to taste.
Combine the dressing and salad mixture.
Let stand at least 30 minutes before serving.
Yields 4 cups

JOE'S SALAD

JOE MORRA, POTLUCKER

We are lucky to have Joe as one of our potluckers.
Joe is a contractor by day and an organic gardener by night.
So when Joe brings a salad, all of the ingredients usually come from his garden.
He is a wealth of information. So whenever I have an organic gardening question, I contact Joe.

Joe was one of our featured speakers at one of our potlucks;
we held it at his gardens and the potluckers had a wonderful time.
Joe uses heirloom seeds which are the best.
I hope this book will help to inspire you to start growing your own food as well.
That way it's local, fresh and better for you.
I hope you will aspire to put energy and love into growing your own crops
and enjoy watching your little baby plants grow each day.
For those of you who are already doing this, you know how rewarding and satisfying it is.

A salad is a living thing and subject to constant change. So in making any salad, follow the axioms
of living food and let your imagination run wild. Below is a sample for a tasty salad.

Prep: 20 minutes

spring mix salad greens

onion

tomatoes

avocados

cucumber

orange and yellow peppers

shredded carrots (zucchini or summer squash also work)

olives

mushrooms lightly coated in raw soy sauce

sea salt

lemon juice

Slice, chop and dice all produce and place in a large bowl.

Then sprinkle with sea salt and lemon juice.

Lemon juice and sea salt are used as a flavoring and an oxidation retardant.

SERGEI'S FAVORITE SALAD
SERGEI & VALYA BOUTENKO, From *EATING WITHOUT HEATING*

Whenever potlucker Karen brings this dish to a potluck it is always a hit.
Check out *Eating Without Heating* by Sergei & Valya Boutenko,
the book contains not only this recipe but other tasty recipes.

Soak Arame: 3 minutes
Prep: 15 minutes

½ cup arame, soaked

1 cup red leaf lettuce, chopped

1 medium tomato, chopped

1 avocado, peeled & diced

1 tablespoon raw tahini

2 tablespoons lemon juice

Soak arame in water for 3 minutes, then drain water. Prepare lettuce, tomato and avocado. Then mix all ingredients in bowl until the tahini is evenly spread throughout the salad.

GINGER HONEY SLAW
ANONYMOUS POTLUCKER

Prep: 15-20 minutes

¾ -1 head green cabbage, chopped
3-5 carrots, grated
ginger, peeled & grated to taste
2 tablespoons sesame seeds (add more if preferred)

Prepare all the ingredients listed above and place in a large bowl. Add dressing.

DRESSING
2-3 tablespoons raw soy sauce
2-3 tablespoons honey

In a small bowl, combine raw soy sauce and honey.
Mix well, then sample for desired taste.
Toss with salad and enjoy.

SUMMERTIME CURRIED CORN SALAD

JANICE INNELLA, THE BEAUTY CHEF, POTLUCKER

Prep Salad: 10 minutes
Prep Dressing: 10 minutes
Prep Mayonnaise: 10 minutes
Marinate Dressing: 2-4 hours

6-8 ears fresh corn or 3 cups frozen corn kernals

1 small zucchini, diced

1 large red bell pepper, diced

1 bunch scallions, white and tender part of green, cut into ¼ inch pieces

½ cup Italian parsley, chopped

In a large bowl, combine the above.

DRESSING

1¼ cup organic, unrefined flax or pumpkin seed oil

4 tablespoons raw organic apple cider vinegar or lemon juice

1 teaspoon curry powder

½ teaspoon sea salt

1-2 garlic cloves, minced

Optional: Add 1-2 tablespoons homemade raw mayonnaise for a creamier dressing.

Mix the dressing ingredients until well blended.

Pour the dressing over the bowl of veggies. Toss and mix well.

Allow combination to marinate for 2 to 4 hours.

MAYONNAISE

1 cup raw cashews

2 young Thai coconuts, meat only

1 lemon, juice

1 teaspoon raw honey

1 teaspoon sea salt

½ cup raw olive oil, cold pressed

⅛ teaspoon cayenne

In a blender, add all ingredients and blend until smooth.

Chill the portion you do not use for later use.

CHINESE BROCCOLI IN GARLIC SOY SAUCE

RAW CHEF DAN, QUINTESSENCE, MANHATTAN

I am pleased to say, I have had the privilege of taking several of Raw Chef Dan's raw cooking classes. I am also honored to call him a friend.
He is a genius in the kitchen. If you ever get to Manhattan,
make sure you stop in and dine at his restaurant Quintessence. It is worth the trip.

Raw Chef Dan made this Chinese Broccoli recipe at a raw buffet
he put on at one of my raw potlucks and then he added Red Pepper Cheese *(p.113)*,
thoroughly coating the broccoli and then heating it in the dehydrator.
It was so tasty; there was no evidence of it on the buffet. It definitely was the hit of the evening.

Prep: 10-15 minutes
Dehydrate: 3 hours at 95 degrees

4 whole dates, pitted

1 cup water

2 tablespoons raw soy sauce (use wheat-free tamari if you are allergic to wheat)

1 large garlic clove

1 inch piece ginger

1 tablespoon raw olive oil

¼ tablespoon sea salt

In a blender combine all ingredients.
Blend until smooth.
Set aside while you prepare the broccoli.

Chinese broccoli

sliced raw almonds

Wash broccoli then place in large bowl.
Pour the blended mixture over broccoli and toss until thoroughly coated.
Place on Teflex liner trays and dehydrate for about 3 hours.
Put in serving bowl and sprinkle with almonds.

This also works well with regular broccoli, choy sum, and bok choy.

HERB PASTA

JOEL ODHNER, PERSONAL CHEF & NUTRITION COACH
This recipe is the first recipe on which I learned how to work a spiralizer.
I must confess I was all thumbs the first time I attempted a spiralizer,
which is comical because it's so easy to use. That is if you know what you are doing.
Luckily, Joel was patient enough to walk me through how it works.
I'm definitely not mechanically inclined! However, this recipe is very easy and deliciously tasty!

Prep: 15-20 minutes
Chill: 1 hour

2-3 medium yams, spiralized, julienned or cut into thin "pasta" slices
½ cup fresh basil, chopped
¼ cup fresh parsley, chopped
⅛-¼ cup raw olive oil
Celtic sea salt to taste

Use a spiralizer to spiralize yams or cut in julienned slices or into thin slices similar to pasta shape.
In a large bowl, combine the yams and the remaining ingredients together.
Chill for one hour in fridge.

Ranch Dill Dressing

JANICE INNELLA, THE BEAUTY CHEF, POTLUCKER
This is great as a dressing or as a topping on veggie burgers or as a dip.

Prep: 15 minutes

1 cup raw cashews
2 young Thai coconuts *(meat only)*
½ cup raw olive oil
1 bunch dill
1 tablespoon light miso
½ teaspoon salt
⅛ red onion
½ cup or more pure water

In a high powered blender, add all of the ingredients and blend until smooth and creamy.

Add more water if the mixture is too thick.

GARDEN BLEND SOUP

CHERIE SORIA, LIVING LIGHT CULINARY INSTITUE OF RAW FOODS IN FORT BRAGG, CA

I have been making this soup ever since I attended
the Living Light Culinary Institute of Raw Foods.
This soup can be made in advance, stored in ball jars and packed in your cooler to eat for lunch.
It is extremely healthy for you and filling, too!

The orange juice gives sweetness to the soup.
For a less sweet soup, reduce or eliminate the orange juice and replace it with additional water.

You can use a variety of vegetables in garden soups such as
cucumbers, zucchini, tomato, bell pepper, celery, kale, and spinach.
Choose from a variety of fresh herbs, too, such as parsley, dill, cilantro, and basil.

Also, when we were taught this recipe in school, we would put it in a soup bowl and then
sprinkle a mixture of finely chopped apple, red pepper and avocado on top.
Not only is it pleasing to the eye, but you are chewing your soup as well, which is good for you.

Prep: 20-30 minutes

1 apple

1 cucumber, seeded and chopped

½ bunch kale (6-10 leaves)

1 green onion, chopped

1 garlic clove, crushed

¼ cup chopped parsley

½ cup chopped cilantro

½ red jalapeno pepper

or a dash of cayenne pepper

2 tablespoons light, mellow miso (chickpea)

1 tablespoon lemon juice

1½ cups water

1 avocado

½ cup orange juice (read above)

Cut the apple in fourths, removing the core and seeds.

In a blender, combine all ingredients except the avocado and blend until smooth.

Now, add the avocado and blend until smooth.

Pour soup in serving bowls.

TOPPING

avocado

apple

red pepper

Finely chop the topping ingredients and sprinkle on top of soup and serve.

REFRESHING CUCUMBER SOUP

RUTH HARP, WHOLE FOODS MARKET, WYNEWOOD, PENNSYLVANIA

This is the recipe for Ruth's favorite cucumber soup.
She said the key is to taste and adjust the ingredients if needed!
Ruth loves this soup because it is so fresh and delicious; she is known to eat it for breakfast.

Use cucumbers from your garden or the following varieties: Kirby, English, or Persian.
If buying from a store, avoid the waxy textured ones.
The goal is to use cucumbers with small and fewer seeds.

You can use the leaves from the celery stalks.
If you are using the outer stalks, they can produce a strong bitter taste,
so you may want to use less.

Prep: 20 minutes

3-6 cucumbers depending on the size

1-2 celery stalks

2 scallions, chopped

⅓ bunch fresh dill, washed; use the stems too!

3 limes juiced (use the pulp too!)

1 small garlic clove, peeled

Real Salt or Braggs Liquid Aminos to taste

¼ -½ fresh jalapeno, as your taste dictates

black pepper to taste

2 tablespoons extra virgin olive oil

2-3 cups filtered or spring water

Wash and trim, but do not peel the cucumbers, then cut into large chunks and place in the blender. Cut the celery stalks into large pieces, and then add to blender. Add the remaining ingredients and blend until smooth. Taste and adjust as needed. Soup will stay fresh for up to 3 days in the fridge.

Add avocado if you want to make your soup richer and thicker or add water to make it lighter and thinner.

Three-Nut Basil Pesto Pasta
Lentil Burgers
Thai Roll Ups with Dipping Sauce
Toona Salad
Pizza with Pizza Sauce & Cheez Topping
Raw Pizza Crust
Chick-un Salad
Maryann's Chili
Atlantic Crab Cakes
Veggie Burger
Sunburgers
Burgers
Vito's Raw Ravioli
Vibrant Veggie Nori Rolls
Sassy Sausages

Some consider dessert to be the climax or the grand event of a meal,
but for me the entree is the most climatic moment of the meal.

When people are new to raw foods, it's always interesting because
everyone says the same thing...
"Everything looks so great. The food is so tasty."
And their final comment,
"The food is so filling. I had no idea raw foods could taste so good."

As you try a few or all of these recipes in this section,
you will amaze your taste buds and be joyously happy.

THREE-NUT BASIL PESTO PASTA

LISA MONTGOMERY

I like to make the pesto and store it in a container and spiralize zucchini and put it in a plastic bag wrapped in a paper towel and store in the fridge.
When I am ready to prepare my meal, it takes only minutes.
By keeping the items separate in storage baggies or containers, it allows everything to stay fresh.

It's also a handy and tasty meal to pack for lunch at work.
It's easy to prepare, I just put the greens in a bowl or plate,
throw on the already spiralized zucchini.
Slice up some asparagus and cherry tomatoes,
chop up cilantro and toss on top of the greens and zucchini.
Then I top with a glob of pesto.

If you are serving this to other people,
you can make it like a buffet and have them build their own meal.
Everyone is different in what they like and don't like,
this way they can create their dish to their own preference.

The sauce alone makes a fabulous dip,
and you can add whatever vegetables you want to the zucchini.

Prep: 10-15 minutes
Prep Pesto: 10 minutes

4 medium zucchini, spiralized
cherry tomatoes, quartered or whole
6 asparagus stalks, thinly sliced on an angle
½ cup chopped fresh cilantro

Use a spiral slicer to cut the zucchini into long strips and put in a serving bowl.
Add the other ingredients to the bowl.

PESTO

2 cups raw pine nuts
½ cup raw cashews
½ cup raw macadamia nuts
4 garlic cloves, minced
6 tablespoons fresh lemon juice
4 teaspoons Himalayan salt
1 cup basil, freshly chopped

In a food processor, combine all the pesto ingredients and process until smooth and sauce-like.
Pour the sauce over the vegetables and toss well.

LENTIL BURGERS

NOMI SHANNON, THE RAW GOURMET

Soak Sunflower Seeds: 8-12 hours
Sprout Sunflower Seeds: 4 hours
Prep: 15-20 minutes
Dehydrate: 8-12 hours

2 cups sunflower seeds, soaked & sprouted
1½ cups sprouted lentils
4 carrots, finely grated
1 small onion, cut in chunks
4 stalks celery, peeled and coarsely chopped
2-3 cloves garlic, chopped
2 scallions, chopped
4 tablespoons chopped parsley
4 tablespoons lemon juice
2 tablespoon liquid aminos or ½ teaspoon sea salt
1 tablespoon poultry seasoning
2 teaspoons fresh oregano or 1 teaspoon dried

In food processor, combine all ingredients.
Process until the ingredients are thoroughly mixed and broken into small bits.
(Depending on the size of your food processor, you may have to process this recipe in batches.)

Form the mixture into ½ inch thick patties.
Dehydrate 8-12 hours or leave them in the sun or warm them in a very low oven.
Makes 9-10 large patties.

THAI ROLL UPS WITH DIPPING SAUCES

JANICE INNELLA, THE BEAUTY CHEF, POTLUCKER

This is another recipe from one of Janice Innella's raw cooking classes.
The presentation can be amazing. Be creative and have fun!

Don't toss out the soaked water from the dried fruit, until after your sauce is complete.

Sprout Sunflower Seeds
Prep Roll Up: 20-30 minutes
Prep Sauce: 10 minutes
Marinate Sauces: 30 minutes before serving

THAI ROLL UP

1 red pepper

1 yellow pepper

1 jicama, sliced in strips

1 zucchini

1 cucumber

1 mango

2 cups sunflower sprouts

1 head asparagus

½ red cabbage, whole leaves

1 head butter lettuce

Slice ingredients and place all ingredients on a platter in a creative presentation.

APRICOT MOOSHU DIPPING SAUCE

½ cup dry apricots, soaked
½ cup yellow Hunza raisins, soaked
½ cup dried cranberries, soaked
1½ tablespoons Umeboshi plum paste
1 shallot

Mix all ingredients in a high speed blender along with enough soaking water to make a creamy, smooth consistency.

ALMOND DIPPING SAUCE

1 cup almond butter

½ cup pure water

4 tablespoons toasted sesame oil
            or pumpkin seed oil

1 teaspoon lime juice

1 teaspoon ginger powder
            or ½ inch fresh peeled or scraped

1 small shallot

1 tablespoon lemon grass

1 red chili

1 tablespoon Umeboshi plum paste

1 tablespoon agave syrup

Mix all of the above ingredients in a high speed blender. Pour sauce in a small bowl.

ASSEMBLE THAI ROLL UP

Take a whole cabbage leaf and spread a spoonful of sauce on the leaf.
Then layer it with slices of veggies and mango.
Sprinkle sunflower sprouts on top slices.
Roll up the ends and eat with your hands.
Or just dip the Roll in the sauces.

TOONA SALAD

MICHELLE SCHULMAN, RAW CHEF, ARNOLD'S WAY, LANDSDALE, PENNSYLVANIA

This mixture will last in the refrigerator covered with plastic wrap for 7-10 days.
Make Toona wraps with nori or Toona sandwhiches on Arnold's bread.
Make Toona salads on a bed of greens.
You can also stuff peppers, tomatoes, and celery sticks with the Toona.

This is a huge batch. You may want to cut recipe in half or even smaller.

Soak Almonds: 4-8 hours
Prep: 15-20 minutes

PATE INGREDIENTS

1 cup soaked almonds
3 cups cashews
1 tablespoons dulse flakes
1 teaspoon kelp powder
2 tablespoons Celtic salt
1-2 ounces of agave syrup
½ cup green olives
½-1 cup celery
¼-½ cup red pepper
⅓-½ red onion
½ teaspoon black pepper (or more to taste)
6 ounces fresh lemon juice
6 ounces or less filtered water
    (add small amount at a time)
Optional: ½ cup olive oil
    (if desired for creaminess)

Place all Pate ingredients, except water, in a food processor with an S blade and begin processing.

When the mixture does not move any longer, begin adding filtered water in small amounts to achieve the desired consistency.
Process the mixture until smooth, or leave it chunky if desired!
The chunks will soften in the mix overnight.

Transfer the mixture to a large mixing bowl and set aside while you prepare the Textured ingredients.

TEXTURE INGREDIENTS

4 (or more) large Bubbies raw pickles
1½ cups celery, chopped
2 cups carrot, shredded
1 cup dill, chopped
¾ cup scallions, chopped
¾ cup parsley, chopped

In the "dirty" food processor,
add Bubbies pickles and chopped celery.
Pulse in food processor.
Make sure you don't chop too fine.

Add to Pate mixture and stir well.
Stir in shredded carrot, dill, scallions and parsley.
Your Toona is ready to serve.

ADJUST TO PLEASE YOUR TASTE BUDS

Taste for saltiness, tartness, sweetness, and spiciness, and adjust.

If the TOONA is bland, add lemon and salt or a few olives.

If it is too salty, add agave syrup.

If it tastes dull, add onion and process again.

PIZZA WITH PIZZA SAUCE & CHEEZ TOPPING

JOEL ODHNER, PERSONAL CHEF & NUTRITION COACH

I just love eating homemade pizza.
Because the crust needs to be prepared in advance,
I usually prepare this recipe a day before serving or in the morning.
While the crust is dehydrating, go ahead and make the sauce and cheez.
Then just store the sauce and cheez in the fridge until the crust is ready.
The time you will wait to eat this tasty meal is worth it!

If you like toppings on your pizza go ahead and add your favorites!
I like to add fresh veggies and herbs.

Soak Flax: 2 hours
Soak Buckwheat Groats: 2 hours
Soak Sunflower Seeds: 4 hours

Prep Crust: 10-15 minutes
Dehydrate: 8-10 hours
Prep Sauce: 10 minutes
Prep Cheez: 10 minutes

CRUST

3 carrots
2-3 garlic cloves
1 tablespoon Italian seasoning
½ cup sundried tomato

In food processor mix all ingredients for about 30 seconds.
Then add:

1½ cups flax, soaked
1 cup buckwheat groats, soaked
1 cup sunflower seeds, soaked

Mix until smooth. Spread the mixture on a Teflex sheet about ⅜ to ½ inch thick. Dehydrate for about 8 to 10 hours, flipping the crust halfway through the drying process. At this time remove the Teflex sheet.

ASSEMBLE

When crust is ready, spread sauce over crust then top with Cheez.

Add your choice of topping(s) to your pizza: fresh veggies and/or herbs.

PIZZA SAUCE

2 cups tomato, chopped
½ cup sundried tomato
¼ cup Italian seasoning
1-2 garlic cloves

In a blender, add all ingredients and blend until smooth. Place in a sealed container until ready to use.

CHEEZ

1½ cups Brazil nuts or macadamia nuts
2 tablespoons lemon juice
1 teaspoon salt
pinch of cayenne
water

In a blender, pour all ingredients in container. Then add water to just cover the nuts. Blend until smooth and creamy. Use a spatula to scrape all the mixture out of the blender container into a sealed container. Store in fridge until ready to use.

RAW PIZZA CRUST

FROM CAROL ALT'S BOOK *THE RAW 50*, PAGE 84

I am sharing this recipe with you because this is the crust I demonstrated on my TV pilot.
It is tasty and easy to make.
If I can make it in front of cameras, you can make it in the quiet of your own kitchen.
Watch the demonstration at www.livingdynamically.com.

Soak Ground Flax Seeds: 2 hours
Soak Almonds: 8-12 hours
Prep: 5-10 minutes
Dehydrate: Overnight

1 cup golden flax seeds

1 cup purified water

2 cups almonds, soaked

2 tablespoons onion, chopped

2 tablespoons fresh thyme, chopped

2 tablespoons fresh rosemary, chopped

2 tablespoons fresh oregano, chopped

Grind the flax seeds finely in a spice or coffee grinder.

Then, soak the ground seeds in 1 cup water until water is completely absorbed, about 2 hours, stirring occasionally.

Place the soaked flax seeds in a food processor with remaining ingredients.

Process until the mixture is finely ground and well mixed.

Form into pizza crusts and dehydrate on Teflex sheets at 105 degrees.

CHICK-UN SALAD

MICHELLE SCHULMAN, RAW CHEF, ARNOLD'S WAY, LANDSDALE, PENNSYLVANIA

I just love this dish. It's great all alone or on a bed of greens.
You can store the uneaten portion in the fridge for later in the day. It will stay fresh for 7-10 days.

After pulling the rosemary leaves from sprigs, don't forget to compost the branches!

Soak Almonds: 2-4 hours
Prep: 15 minutes

CHICK-UN SALAD
TEXTURE INGREDIENTS

1 cup almonds, soaked

2 cups cashews

1 cup celery

⅓ purple onion

½ cup red pepper

2 level tablespoons Celtic salt

½ teaspoon or more of black pepper

6 oz fresh lemon juice

1-2 ounces agave syrup

3 or more springs fresh rosemary, to taste

1 teaspoon marjoram & ½ teaspoon thyme
     or 1½ teaspoons poultry seasoning

6 ounces or less filtered water
   (add in small amounts)

optional: ½ cup olive oil

In a food processor with a S blade add ingredients.
Add a small portion of water at a time and blend until mixture achieves desired consistency.
Check for taste and adjust.
Transfer mixture to large bowl.

STEP 2

1½ cups celery, chopped

In "dirty" food processor, pulse chopped celery for 4-5 minutes.
Add celery to Textured mixture.

Add the following to large bowl:

¼ cup parsley, chopped

½ cup scallion, chopped

½ cup red pepper, chopped

Mix thoroughly and serve over a bed of greens or store in airtight container in fridge.
It will last for 7-10 days.

MARYANN'S CHILI

MARYANN O'BRIEN, POTLUCKER

This is the best chili recipe. It is to die for!
People don't realize whether the dish is raw or standard American.
You will adore this recipe and what makes it even better, is that it is good for you.
People always ask, "How long will this dish keep?"
This is another dish where you will eat it up before it spoils.
Frankly, you will eat up all the recipes in this book long before they spoil!

If dates are hard, soak until soft, but not mushy.

Prep: 15-20 minutes

4 tomatoes

2 avocados

½ cup sundried tomatoes

2 teaspoons salt

2 tablespoons chili powder

2 teaspoons ground cumin

In food processor, blend all the ingredients listed above until smooth.
Set aside.

½ cup celery

½ cup carrots

½ cup leeks

1 red pepper

¼ cup olive oil

1 teaspoon salt

Chop the veggies.
Then allow chopped veggies to marinate in olive oil and 1 teaspoon salt for a few minutes.
In a large bowl, combine the processed mixture and the marinated mixture.
Ready to serve.

ATLANTIC CRAB CAKES

RAW CHEF DAN OF QUINTESSENCE, MANHATTAN

If you are in a hurry, you can sprout sunflower seeds for one day.
However, you need to rinse the seeds several times each day!

Sprout Sunflower Seeds: 1-3 days (rinse several times each day)
Prep Butternut Pulp: 15 minutes
Prep: 10 minutes
Dehydrate: 5 hours

½ cup butternut squash pulp from juicer
½ cup sprouted sunflower seeds
½ cup pine nuts
¼ cup dried coconut flakes
1 tablespoon fresh rosemary, finely chopped
1 tablespoon fresh dill, finely chopped
1 teaspoon sea salt
¼ cup dulse (loose)
2 tablespoons lemon juice

Juice a butternut squash. Take ½ cup of the pulp and set aside for this recipe.

Put the remainder of the ingredients into a food processor and mix until well blended.
You will still be able to see the different textured ingredients.
Transfer the mixture to a mixing bowl.

Kneed the butternut squash pulp with a fork or hand.

Form mixture into patties, 2 to 2½ inches wide, and place on a Teflex lined dehydrator sheet.
Dehydrate at 100 degrees for two hours, then flip patties over and remove the Teflex sheet.
Dehydrate another three hours. Serve warm.

Excellent with Tartar Sauce.

TARTER SAUCE
In a bowl, mix 1 cup mayonnaise *(p.136)* with ¼ cup sweet pickle relish.

VEGGIE BURGER

ANONYMOUS POTLUCKER

Soak Almonds: 12-24 hours
Soak Sunflower & Sesame Seeds: 5-6 hours
Prep: 15 minutes
Dehydrate: 12-17 hours

1 large red onion
1 large bell pepper
3 carrots
1 small head cauliflower
1 large stalk broccoli
1 cup almonds, soaked
1 cup sunflower seeds, soaked
¼ cup sesame seeds, soaked
5 garlic cloves
2 tablespoons Braggs or to taste
1 teaspoon cumin
1 tablespoon dried cilantro
    or 1-2 cups fresh cilantro

Blend all of the above ingredients in a food processor or a juicer with a blank plate. This blended mixture is the patty mixture.

Form and place ½" thick patties on Teflex sheets and place trays in the dehydrator. Dehydrate at 105 degrees for 8 to 12 hours or until the desired texture is obtained.

Flip your burgers after 4 hours and remove the Teflex sheets. Continue to dehydrate for 4 to 5 hours or until desired moisture is obtained.

SUNBURGERS

JOEL ODHNER, PERSONAL CHEF & NUTRITION COACH

Soak Almonds & Sunflower Seeds: 2-4 hours
Prep: 20 minutes
Dehydrate: 4-5 hours or until desired firmness

1 pound nuts, soaked

¼ -½ cup flaxseed, ground

1 pound carrots

½ medium onion, diced

2-3 stalks celery, diced

½ pepper, diced

Celtic sea salt to taste

Bragg liquid aminos to taste (optional)

Grind nuts and flaxseeds in blender or food processor. Set aside in large bowl.

Grind carrots in food processor until fine.

Add remaining ingredients.

Form into patties.

Eat as is or dehydrate until desired firmness.

Top with slice of tomato and onion.

Enjoy often!

BURGERS

MODIFICATION FROM JOEL ODHNER'S ORIGINAL RECIPE

A Potlucker brought these to one of our monthly raw potlucks and they were delicious. He used Joel Odhner's original recipe to apply a few twists.

Use a ¼ cup measuring cup to form round patties or a circle cookie cutter.

Soak Almonds & Sunflower Seeds: 2-4 hours
Prep: 20 minutes
Dehydrate: 4-5 hours or until desired firmness

1 cup almonds, soaked
1 cup sunflower seeds, soaked

3 carrots
3 celery stalks
½ red onion
¼ cup chopped parsley
1 cup golden flax, ground
½ cup water

¼ cup olive oil
salt and pepper to taste
parsley to taste

Soak almonds and sunflower seeds for 2-4 hours.
After soaking, grind almonds and sunflower seeds in food processor, then set aside in large bowl.
Grind veggies and add to large bowl.
Add ground flax and water to bowl and mix well.
Take ¼ of mixture and put back in food processor.
While the processor is running, add olive oil.
Return processed mixture to bowl and mix in salt, pepper and parsley.
Form mixture into patties and dehydrate to desired firmness.
Dehydrate at 140 for 30 minutes on Teflex sheets.
After 30 minutes, flip them and put them directly on rack.
Turn dehydrator down to 115 degrees for 4 to 5 hours.

VITO'S RAW RAVIOLI

VITO NATALE, POTLUCKER

I have made this ravioli dish numerous times and I never tire of it.

Mandolin Turnips: 15 minutes
Prep Cheese Filling: 10 minutes
Prep Marinara Sauce: 10 minutes
Assemble: 10 minutes

PASTA WRAPPER

4 turnips

Wash the turnips and cut in half.
Use a mandolin to make paper thin slices
that you can fold.
These will be used for the outside
of the ravioli.

CHEESE FILLING

1 cup pine nuts
½ cup macadamia nuts or cashews
1 cup walnuts
8 teaspoons lemon juice
6 teaspoons Bragg liquid aminos
2 garlic cloves
1 teaspoon cilantro, fresh
1 pinch oregano

In a food processor or blender,
add all the cheese filling ingredients
and blend until creamy.
Place the cheese filling
in a bowl and set aside.

MARINARA SAUCE

2 cups tomatoes
12 sundried tomatoes, soaked
3 dates, soaked & pitted
¼ cup olive oil
1 teaspoon apple cider vinegar
2 teaspoons raw honey
4 garlic cloves
2 tablespoons parsley
1 teaspoon sea salt
⅛ teaspoon cayenne
1 teaspoon black pepper
1 teaspoon basil, fresh (or to taste)
1 teaspoon oregano, fresh

In same processor or blender, combine all the
marinara sauce ingredients and blend well.

ASSEMBLE

Take one slice of turnip at a time and add a
spoonful of cheese to center.
Fold the turnip in half to form a half circle and
place on a dish.
Do this until you have about 10 on a dish.
Then drizzle the marinara sauce over
the ravioli. Let sit for a few hours or serve.
Optional: Sprinkle raw cheese on top.

VIBRANT VEGGIE NORI ROLLS

RECIPE FROM TONYA ZAVASTA'S, *BEAUTIFUL ON RAW: UNCOOKED CREATIONS*

Grace brought this to one of the potlucks and it was absolutely tasty.
A quick way to dehydrate sunflower seeds is to put them in the dehydrator for 2-4 hours.

Soak Almonds: Overnight
Soak Sunflower Seeds: Overnight
Dehydrate Sunflower Seeds: 2-4 hours
Prep: 15 minutes

2 cups almonds, soaked & rinsed

1 medium bell pepper, cut in chunks

Sea salt to taste

½ cup sunflower seeds, soaked, rinsed & dried (no shells)

1 celery stalk, finely minced

10 raw nori sheets (sun-dried)

2 large carrots, spiralized or cut in long strips

1 large beet, spiralized or shredded

2 avocados cut in long strips

10 green onions, sliced in half lengthwise

1 cup alfalfa sprouts

Soak almonds and sunflower seeds in separate bowls overnight.
Combine almonds, bell pepper chunks, and sea salt in a food processor.
Process until smooth paste is formed.
Remove the mixture from the food processor and place in a bowl.
Stir in sunflower seeds, and minced celery. Mix well with a spoon.

Spread the mixture about 1 inch wide and ¼ inch thick along the short side of a nori sheet.
On the same side, layer with prepared carrots, beets, avocado strips, green onion, and alfalfa sprouts.

Starting with the edge closest to you, using both hands, gently roll each nori into a log.
Moisten the outer edge of the nori with water to help seal it.
Repeat procedure for all nori rolls.
Cut the rolls into cylinders 1 inch long. Serve.

SASSY SAUSAGES

PEGGY O'NEIL, POTLUCKER

Soak Walnuts: 2-4 hours
Dehydrate Walnuts: 4 hours
Prep: 20-30 minutes
Dehydrate: 5 hours

3 cups walnut pieces, soaked & dried

1 small beet

½ white onion

2 medium carrots

2 garlic cloves

2 tablespoons agave syrup

2 tablespoons Nama Shoyu

1 teaspoon A-1 steak sauce *(Note: this is not a raw food!)*

1 teaspoon marjoram

1 teaspoon celery salt

1 teaspoon paprika

Soak walnuts in water for 2-4 hours. Then dehydrate until dry.

In a food processor, combine all ingredients and blend to desired consistency.
Depending on the size of your food processor, you may have to process in several batches and
then mix all the batches together in one bowl.

Extrude (process the mixture through the juicer) using a juicer with a blank blade
to form ½ x 3-inch "sausages" or shape into patties by hand.
Dehydrate about five hours.
Makes about 45 "sausages."

BERRIES & CREAM
CHOCOLATE MOUSSE WITH RASPBERRY CREAM
BANANA CREPE ROLL
CHOCOLATE MOUSSE PIE
BLUEBERRY CREAM PIE
COCONUT CREAM PIE
CHOCOLATE FUDGE
PECAN PIE
COCONUT RASPBERRY BLISS BALLS
SWEET CASHEW CREAM
TRIFLE TART
JUICY PEAR TART
LEMON DREAM PIE
SQUASH PIE
VITO'S APPLE PIE
VITO'S BROWNIES
VITO'S FROZEN WATERMELON CHEESECAKE
PECAN DREAM PIE
FRUIT & CHOCOLATE DECADENCE

After smoothies, I would say the next easiest way
for a person to go raw is desserts.
Everyone loves desserts.
Raw desserts not only are beautiful and tasty, they are nutritious.
If you take a raw dessert to a party and don't tell the guests it is raw,
your raw dessert will most likely be the first dessert to be eaten up.
After the dessert has been consumed, then tell them it was raw.
That's usually when their response is,
"No way!...I thought raw food was carrot sticks."
Again, another raw food myth busted.

D
E
S
S
E
R
T
S

If you are not up to making your own desserts and sweet treats
and you don't live in the Philadelphia suburbs...Never fear!
Tiffany Watts, who owns a raw restaurant,
"Oasis" in Frazer, Pennsylvania does mail orders.
Her website is www.OasisLivingCuisine.com.
Place an order online or call 877-913-9797.
Tiffany's raw restaurant is truly an oasis.
Yes, you can have a complete raw meal at Oasis,
however her raw chocolate covered pretzels, thumb print cookies
and macaroons are delectable.
I purchase these treats and keep them in the refrigerator.
I think they are better chilled...reminds me of
frozen Milky Way bars when I was young.

BERRIES & CREAM

DEBORAH ROCKWELL, POTLUCKER

You can use other berries that are in season. The more colorful the better.
This dessert is so beautiful to the eye when it is prepared in a glass bowl.
It's so easy to prepare. Your guests will think you spent hours in the kitchen.

Soak Nuts: 2 hours minimum
Prep: 10 -15 minutes

CREAM
4 cups almonds or walnuts, soaked
almond extract, couple of drops
1 cup or more of fresh squeezed orange juice

In a high powdered blender, blend the above ingredients until smooth.
Set aside in fridge until ready to use.

BERRIES
6 cups strawberries, leave about 6 to 8 whole for your garnish
1 cup raspberries
1 cup blueberries

Slice strawberries and remember to save some for a garnish.

Place a layer of strawberries on the bottom of a bowl,
then spread a layer of cream over the strawberries.

Continue to layer fruit, and then top with cream.

The last layer should have a mixture of berries displayed beautifully.

Garnish with fresh mint leaves and whole strawberries.

CHOCOLATE MOUSSE WITH RASPBERRY CREAM

KATHERYN JENSEN, POTLUCKER

This dessert is yummy. Children of all ages also enjoy this chocolate treat.
Don't tell them about the avocados, just let them enjoy.
What I love about this tasty treat is it will last in my fridge for days,
that is if I don't eat it all in one day!

If you add too much date water to mixture, the consistency of the mousse and cream will be too runny. It will still taste yummy, but it will not look pleasing to your guests.
So be on the safe side and add a little date water at a time until the mixture is creamy.

Soak Dates: 15 minutes (save water from soaking)

Soak Cashews: 30 minutes

Prep: 30 minutes

Chill: 1-2 hours (or eat not chilled...you may not be able to wait!)

CHOCOLATE MOUSSE (makes 5 cups)

5 avocados, ripe

1¼ cups dates, pitted plus 8 more, soaked

3 tablespoons alcohol free vanilla extract

2 tablespoons coconut oil,
cold pressed extra virgin

1 teaspoon sea salt

2 tablespoons pure maple syrup

3 tablespoons raw honey

1½ cups raw cocoa

Optional: raw walnuts, chopped

Soak dates for 15 minutes.
Drain and save water. Set aside.

Put all ingredients in food processor or high powered blender. Blend until very smooth, thick and creamy. You will have to add a few tablespoons of the date water a little at a time while blending.

Spread mixture in a serving dish such as a pie dish or in individual bowls. Place in the fridge while you prepare the cream.
It will keep for several days in the fridge.

RASPBERRY CREAM

2 cups raw cashews, soaked

8-12 large soft dates or 12-16 small dates,
pitted & soaked

2 tablespoons raw honey

2 tablespoons coconut oil,
cold pressed extra virgin

2 tablespoons alcohol free vanilla extract

½ cup raspberries, fresh or thawed frozen

Soak cashews in 1½ cups water for 30 minutes. Drain and rinse. Soak dates in ½ cup water until very moist. Drain and be sure to save the date water.
In a high powered blender, blend all ingredients. Adding date water, if needed, a little at a time. Blend until smooth.

TO ASSEMBLE

Spread the Raspberry Cream on top of the Chocolate Mousse.

OPTIONAL: Garnish with chopped raw walnuts around the edges. Keep in refrigerator until ready to serve.

BANANA CREPE ROLL

LINDA COOPER, POTLUCKER

This crepe is delicious and can be made with a variety of fillings.
You may find a favorite filling from one of the recipes below.

Crepes can be made ahead and frozen until ready for use.

Soak Dried Apricots: Overnight
Soak Dates: 20 minutes
Prep Bananas: Less than 10 minutes
Dehydrate Bananas: 18 to 24 hours
Prep Filling: 30 minutes

BANANA CREPE

5-6 ripe bananas

Blend bananas in a food processor and spread evenly on a Teflex sheet.
To prevent sticking, spread a bit of coconut or olive oil on Teflex sheet before spreading banana puree.
Dehydrate at 95 degrees for 18 to 24 hours.
Prepare one of the fillings.

NUT CREAM FILLING

1 cup macadamia nuts
1 cup cashews
1 teaspoon lemon juice
2 tablespoons agave syrup(to taste)
1 teaspoon vanilla
Water
Optional:
Dash of cinnamon and vanilla powder

Put all ingredients in a high powered blender and blend until smooth and creamy.
Add water a little at a time until mixture turns into a thick cream.
Set aside until ready to assemble crepe.

APRICOT BANANA PUDDING FILLING

1 cup dried apricots, soaked & drained
2 bananas
8 dates, soaked & drained
1 teaspoon vanilla extract
¼ cup raw almond butter

In a food processor, blend all ingredients into a puree. Set aside until ready to assemble crepe.

RASPBERRY STRAWBERRY SAUCE TOPPING

1 -10 oz. bag frozen organic raspberries
½-¾ -10 oz. bag frozen organic strawberries
½ cup dates

Blend ingredients in food processor until smooth.
Set aside until ready to assemble crepe.

ASSEMBLE CREPE

After bananas are dehydrated, peel the banana crepe from Teflex sheet. It is best to use the exposed side of the crepe as the inside of the crepe. Place the banana crepe on a smooth, clean surface. Then spread the filling on the banana crepe and roll up evenly.
Place on a serving dish and then drizzle the Raspberry Strawberry Sauce on top.

CHOCOLATE MOUSSE PIE

JOEL ODHNER, PERSONAL CHEF & NUTRITION COACH

This is another simple and tasty recipe and no one will ever guess there are avocados in it.
You can just make the filling and serve it in pretty little pudding/custard cups
and garnish with slices of fresh strawberries and a piece of mint.

I also love the fact that this mousse will last five to seven days in the fridge,
that is if you don't eat it all by then!

Joel's kids even eat this for breakfast and dinner on the same day.
Why not, it's so healthy and delicious!

Prep: 15 minutes
Chill: 1 hour (or not!)

CRUST

2 cups shredded coconut

2 cups dates, pitted

Place the shredded coconut in a food
processor for about 30 seconds,
then add the dates and process until sticky.
Press mixture into pie plate.

FILLING

2-3 ripe avocados

½ cup coconut oil

¾ cup agave syrup

1 cup cacao powder

Put all the ingredients in a food processor
and blend until smooth.
Pour filling into the crust and chill for 1 hour.

BLUEBERRY CREAM PIE

JOEL ODHNER, PERSONAL CHEF & NUTRITION COACH

This is another recipe where I have been known to make the crust in advance and freeze it just because I knew I wouldn't have time the day of the event.

I've also frozen the crust and taken it on RV trips with my parents
and then all I need to make is the filling and assemble the pie.
So that's how easy it is, even in a small kitchen of a RV you can still put together a fabulous pie.

This pie will last 3 to 5 days refrigerated, that is unless you haven't eaten it all up.

Prep Crust: 5 minutes
Prep Filling: 5 minutes
Chill: 1-2 hours before serving

CRUST

2 cups shredded coconut
1½-2 cups dates, pitted

Place shredded coconut in food processor for about 30 seconds.
Then add dates and process until sticky.
Press mixture into pie pan.

FILLING

2 cups blueberries
1½ cups young, Thai coconut meat
2 tablespoons coconut oil
½ teaspoon cinnamon

Process all ingredients in food processor until smooth.
Pour filling into pie crust.
Chill for 1 hour.

COCONUT CREAM PIE

Joel Odhner, Personal Chef & nutrition Coach

I have been known to make the pie crust in advance and just freeze it,
so it's ready to go when I need to make a dessert fast.
This is a very simple recipe. Just because this recipe is uncomplicated, though,
don't diminish how good it will taste.

I never used to like coconuts before I went raw. Now, I adore them.
So, even if you aren't a coconut fan, you may find this recipe amazing.
Oh by the way, did I tell you how good coconuts are for you?
What more could you ask for: healthy and tasty. Now, that's a win-win. Thank you, Joel!

Prep Crust: 5-10 minutes
Prep Filling: 5-10 minutes
Chill: 1 hour

CRUST

2 cups shredded coconut

1-2 cups dates, pitted

Place shredded coconut in food processor
for about 30 seconds.

Then add dates and process until sticky.
Press mixture into a pie plate.

FILLING

2 young Thai coconuts, meat

Coconut water for consistency (from coconuts)

1 cup shredded coconut

¼ cup coconut oil

2 tablespoons agave syrup

Pinch of nutmeg

Pinch of sea salt

Blend all ingredients in blender until smooth.
Pour into pie crust.
Chill for 1 hour.

CHOCOLATE FUDGE

Dawn Light, From *Dawn of a New Day Desserts*, potlucker

I prefer to use wax paper when preparing fudge pieces.
As I press the mixture between two pieces of wax paper,
my hands stay clean and the mixture forms a smooth surface.
You can also use a rolling pin to spread the fudge...
just remember to put the fudge mixture between two large pieces of wax paper.

Hint: If dates are hard, soak until soft but not mushy.

Soak Cacao Nibs: 1 hour
Dry Cacao Nibs: Until dry
Prep: 15 minutes
Chill: 1–2 hours

2 cups raw cacao nibs, soaked & dried
2½ cups or 20 dates

Soak cacao nibs for one hour, then set aside to dry or place in a dehydrator.
Pitt dates, and then blend in food processor until smooth. Remove from processor and set aside.

In a food processor, blend cacao nibs, scrapping sides of bowl frequently,
until the nibs become liquid.

Monitor the temperature so the mixture does not get hotter than 105 degrees while blending.
If it gets too hot, stop blending and let it cool before continuing.

Add blended dates to cacao mixture and blend thoroughly scraping the sides of the bowl
as needed.

Press mixture between 2 pieces of wax paper until ½ or ¾ inch thick, depending on your
preference. Or roll a rolling pin over the wax paper to make the fudge smooth.

Refrigerate until solid.

Cut into bite size pieces and store in the refrigerator.
Makes about 20 pieces.
Serve chilled.

PECAN PIE

TIONA BROWN, POTLUCKER

Tiona's recipes are always amazing and they will blow you away.
I keep telling Tiona that she could have her own restaurant and the place would be packed.
Her dishes always look great and taste delicious.

Soak Almonds: 4-6 hours
Soak Dates: 30 minutes
Prep Crust: 10 minutes
Prep Filling: 10 minutes

PIE CRUST

2 cups almonds, soaked

6-10 dates, pitted & soaked

½ teaspoon vanilla (alcohol-free)

Dash of cinnamon

2 teaspoons water or 1 teaspoon maple syrup

Soak almonds then allow time for them to dry.

Chop the dates.

Then, combine all of the above ingredients in a food processor. Blend thoroughly.

Pack mixture into serving dish to form crust.

PECAN PIE FILLING

2 cups raw pecans

4-6 dates, pitted & soaked

½ teaspoon vanilla

2 teaspoons water

dash cinnamon

First, grind the pecans in the food processor.

Then, blend all ingredients in food processor.

For a smoother filling, add more water.

For a sweeter taste, add a dash of maple syrup.

Pour filling into crust and refrigerate.

COCONUT RASPBERRY BLISS BALLS

TIONA BROWN, POTLUCKER

These bliss balls are simply the almond crust mixture from Tiona's Pecan Pie recipe.

This dish was made especially for me at one of my potlucks. I was so honored.
You will absolutely adore these.
Whenever you want a berry bliss treat, grab a berry ball from your freezer!

Pie Crust Recipe (p. 166): 10 minutes
Prep: 30 minutes
Soak balls: 4-6 hours

ALMOND BALLS

Pie Crust mixture from the Pecan Pie recipe on page 166

Use leftover pie crust mixture or make the entire batch,
so you will have more mixture to make more Bliss Balls.
Take the pie crust mixture and form bite size balls.

RASPBERRY SAUCE

1 cup fresh raspberries (or defrost a bit first, if frozen)
⅓ cup agave syrup

In a bowl, use a hand blender to blend raspberries and agave syrup.
Then soak the balls in the bowl of raspberry sauce for 4-6 hours.

COCONUT COATING

raw coconut flakes (depends on how many balls you make)

Place shredded coconut in a sandwich size plastic bag.
Then toss the soaked balls in the bag with coconut flakes.
Simply coat the balls, and remove the balls from the bag.

Take a bite and enjoy.
Store uneaten balls in fridge or freezer.

SWEET CASHEW CREAM

BROUGHT BY DEBORAH ROCKWELL, POTLUCKER

(Recipe is from The Raw Revolution Diet by Cherie Soria, page 107)

This is a very simple recipe to make. It looks great and is absolutely delectable.
Serve with a fruit salad, berries, or fruit of your choice.
Or add a glob on a chocolate brownie.

Soak Cashews: 2-4 hours
Prep: 5 minutes
Chill: 1 hour

¼ cup dates, pitted or agave syrup

1 cup cashews, soaked

½ cup purified water

Soak cashews in water for 2-4 hours.

After soaking, be sure to drain and rinse cashews.

Loosely separate dates and place them in a blender with cashews and water.

Process until smooth, adding more water to thin if necessary.

Chill in a sealed glass jar in the refrigerator for at least 1 hour.

It will keep for up to 1 week.

TRIFLE TART

JANICE INNELLA, THE BEAUTY CHEF, POTLUCKER

This is another one of my favorites. Okay, I have many favorites.
However, it is one of the best desserts I have ever eaten. It is amazing!

You will need a large glass bowl or trifle dish to display this dessert.

Soak Cherries: 30 minutes or until softened

Prep: 20 minutes

Chill: 20 minutes

2 cups dry cherries, soaked in pure water

4 kiwi (peel & slice)

2 cups cashews

1 raw vanilla bean

⅛ teaspoon Celtic sea salt

2 tablespoons honey

1 pint blueberries

1 pint raspberries

2 cups raw pistachios

2 tablespoons agave syrup

In a small bowl, place 2 cups dry cherries and cover with water.
Allow to soak for about 30 minutes or until softened.
In a high speed blender, blend cherries with water until smooth.
Pour cherry mixture in a glass bowl or trifle dish.

Place sliced kiwi on top of cherry mixture.

In blender, blend cashews, vanilla bean, pinch of salt and raw honey until smooth.
Pour on top of kiwi slices.

Decorate top of cashew mixture with blueberries.
In blender, blend raspberries and drizzle into middle of bowl.

Pulse pistachios in a food processor with agave syrup.
Decorate around bowl. Chill until ready to serve.

JUICY PEAR TART

POTLUCKER MYRRIAH JANNETTE, FORMER OWNER OF RAW FOOD CAFÉ *LUNA PASTEL*

I just love the candied walnuts on top of this tart.
So, I prepare the walnuts before I begin making the tart.

Prep Candied Walnuts: Soak 4 hours then dehydrate till dry
Soak Walnuts: Overnight
Soak Raisins: 1 hour
Soak Cashews: 4 hours
Prep Crust: 5-10 minutes
Prep Pears: 5-10 minutes
Prep Whipped Creme: 5-10 minutes
Chill: Overnight

CANDIED WALNUTS

1½ cup chopped walnuts, soaked & drained
agave syrup

In a mixing bowl, combine walnuts and agave
syrup. Spread on Teflex sheet.
Dehydrate on 105 degrees until dry.
These will be used as the topping.

CRUST

2 cups walnuts, soaked, rinsed & drained
1 cup raisins, soaked in warm water,
        rinsed & drained

Soak walnuts for 4 hours, then rinse and drain.
Soak raisins in warm water for one hour,
then rinse and drain.
Blend ingredients in food processor.

Line a bottom of 9-inch spring form cake pan
with wax paper. Form the crust mixture to the
bottom of the cake pan.

PEAR MIXTURE FILLING

4 cups grated pears
2 tablespoons lemon juice
1 tablespoon cinnamon
¼ teaspoon nutmeg
⅓ cup agave
4 teaspoons psyllium

In a large bowl, combine all ingredients and
mix well. Then spread mixture on top of
crust.

WHIPPED CREME

1 cup cashews, soaked & well drained
½ cup Thai coconut water
5 dates, soaked in warm water until soft,
        drain well
1 tablespoon coconut butter

Blend all ingredients in blender until smooth.
Spread over pear mixture.
Sprinkle with Candied Walnuts on top of
creme. Refrigerate overnight before serving.

LEMON DREAM PIE

Janice Innella, The Beauty Chef, Potlucker

This recipe is a dream!

Prep: 30 minutes
Freeze: 1 or more hours

4 young Thai coconuts, meat only
½ cup coconut juice, from young Thai coconut
1 cup cashews
½ cup coconut oil
⅛ teaspoon Celtic sea salt
lemon zest from 4 lemons
2 tablespoons lemon juice
4 tablespoons raw honey
1 inch grated ginger
1 teaspoon maca

Crack open the coconut and harvest the meat and juice.
In a high powered blender, add all ingredients and blend until creamy.
Pour the mixture in a pie dish.

GARNISH
2 tablespoons dry coconut
½ cup pecans, chopped
lemon zest

Garnish with lemon zest, pecans and dry coconut. Freeze for one hour or more.
Serve with lemon balm leaves.

SQUASH PIE

TIONA BROWN, POTLUCKER

Tiona's recipes are always amazing and they will blow you away.
I keep telling Tiona that she could have her own restaurant and the place would be packed.
Her dishes always look great and taste delicious.

Soak Dates: 30 minutes
Prep: 20 minutes

1 Kibachi squash or two small acorn squash
6 dates, soaked & pitted
Dash of cinnamon
½ teaspoon vanilla

Remove pitts from dates.
Then soak dates in water for 30 minutes.

While dates are soaking, peel skin from squash and remove all seeds.

Put the dates and the squash through a juicer.
You may have to do this twice if the squash does not have a smooth consistency.

Place all remaining ingredients and squash mixture in a food processor and run until smooth.

If the mixture is not sweet enough for you,
consider adding 1 to 2 teaspoons of agave or maple syrup.

VITO'S APPLE PIE
VITO NATALE, POTLUCKER

Prep Crust: 5 minutes
Prep Filling: 15 minutes

CRUST

1½ cups sunflower seeds

¾ cup raisins

1 tablespoon raw carob powder

Process all the crust ingredients in a food processor then pat in a 9-inch pie plate.

FILLING

5-6 medium size apples, peeled & cored

¾ cup raw honey with bee pollen

1 tablespoon cinnamon

Juice from ½ lemon

Dash of clove

1 small banana

handful of raisins

pinch of sea salt

Optional: shredded coconut

Put all the filling ingredients in a food processor and blend until small chunks form.
Scoop the mixture into a pie plate over the crust.
Sprinkle shredded coconut on top of the pie.

VITO'S BROWNIES

VITO NATALE, POTLUCKER

Prep: 10 minutes
Dehydrate: 6-8 hours

2 cups shredded dried coconut

2 Medjool dates, pitted

3 tablespoons raw honey

1 tablespoon carob powder

1 teaspoon vanilla extract

Blend all the ingredients thoroughly in a blender or food processor
until finely chopped and well combined.

With your hands, form the mixture into 2 x 4 inch rectangles, each about ¾ inch thick.
If they don't hold together, add a bit more honey to the mixture.

Place the brownies on Teflex lined dehydrator trays and
dehydrate at 105 degrees for 6 to 8 hours, depending on how moist you like them.

VITO'S FROZEN WATERMELON CHEESECAKE

VITO NATALE, POTLUCKER

I love watermelon and I love cheesecake.
Vito has come up with a winning combo.
Vito is one of the most innovative raw chefs I know.
I just recently found out besides being a raw chef, photographer and video photographer,
he is also a singer!

Prep: 10-15 minutes
Freeze: 1 hour or until firm

1 young Thai coconut

2 cups raw cashews

2 tablespoons agave syrup

2 tablespoons raw honey

pinch of Himalayan salt

1 teaspoon raw sesame seeds

¼ cup water

1 cup watermelon, cubed & seeded

Optional for topping & garnish:
½ cup almonds, chopped
kiwi slices

Open the coconut. You will need ½ cup coconut water and ¼ cup coconut meat.
Save the rest for something else or make another batch of this recipe.

In a blender or food processor, combine the coconut water and meat with
the remaining ingredients.
Blend until thoroughly combined.

Scrape the mixture into a glass pie dish and place in the freezer for at least 1 hour or until firm.

When ready to serve, cut into wedges and garnish each piece
with a sprinkle of chopped almonds and kiwi slices.

PECAN DREAM PIE

JANICE INNELLA, THE BEAUTY CHEF, POTLUCKER

Another yummy dream creation from Janice

Soak Pecans: 1 hour
Soak Dates: 30 minutes
Prep Crust: 10 minutes
Prep Filling: 10 minutes
Prep Topping: 5 minutes
Freeze Pie: 1 hour
Prep Sauce: 5-10 minutes

CRUST

2 cups pecans
1½ cups dry coconut
½ cup coconut oil
½ teaspoon Celtic Sea Salt
½ cup agave syrup
1 pound raw cacao powder

Blend crust ingredients in food processor.
Press crust mixture into medium size spring form pan. Freeze while you start the other two layers.

FILLING

2 cups pecans, soaked
2 vanilla beans,
split open & scrape out meat with small knife
2 young Thai coconuts (meat only)
½ cup coconut water
4 tablespoons agave syrup
pinch sea salt
½ cup coconut oil

Blend the filling ingredients together
in a high speed blender.
Pour into pan on top of crust.
Sprinkle cacao powder on top of the filling layer.

PECAN TOPPING

1½ cups pecans
1 tablespoon cacao powder
2 tablespoons agave syrup

Chop pecans in food processor and then blend with cacao powder and agave syrup in blender. Sprinkle mixture on top of the pie. Freeze for 1 hour.

CASHEW VANILLA SAUCE
optional

1 cup raw cashews
3 tablespoons agave syrup
1 vanilla bean (meat)
pinch of sea salt
6 tablespoons coconut water
   or 6 tablespoons purified water

Blend all ingredients in high speed blender.
Pour into small container and chill until ready to serve.
Drizzle sauce on top of pie or serve separately.

FRUIT & CHOCOLATE DECADENCE

Vito Natale, Potlucker

Freeze Peeled Bananas: Until frozen
Prep Chocolate & Cashew Cream: 15 minutes
Chill: 1 hour or more
Prep Banana Whip: 5 minutes

1 cup chocolate (chocolate powder made from cacao nibs)

1 cup agave syrup

1 cup raw carob powder

¾ cup coconut oil

1 tablespoon raw sesame seeds

1 handful raw almonds

Blend the above in a food processor until smooth.
Let sit while you make cashew cream in a blender.

Cashew Cream

1 cup cashews

1 cup water

In a blender, blend the cashews and water until smooth.
Add the chocolate mix to the cashew cream and pulsate until smooth.
Spread mixture in a serving dish.
Refrigerate for an hour or more.
Cut into serving pieces and garnish with fresh strawberries, mint leaves and a scoop of banana whip.

Banana Whip

Frozen bananas

Run frozen bananas through juicer using blank blade.
Banana whip in itself is a great dessert.

Index

T

V

W

Z